THE FIRST ANESTHETIC

The Story of Crawford Long

By
FRANK KELLS BOLAND, M.D.

UNIVERSITY OF GEORGIA PRESS
ATHENS

Paperback edition, 2009
© 1950 by the University of Georgia Press
Athens, Georgia 30602
www.ugapress.org
All rights reserved
Printed digitally in the United States of America

The Library of Congress has cataloged the hardcover edition of this book as follows:
Library of Congress Cataloging-in-Publication Data

Boland, Frank Kells.
The first anesthetic;
xv, 160 p. illus., ports., map, facsims. 23 cm.
1. Long, Crawford Williamson, 1815–1878. 2. Anesthetics—History.
3. Ether–History. I. Title.
RD80.L9 B6
50-7365

PAPERBACK ISBN-13: 978-0-8203-3436-3
ISBN-10: 0-8203-3436-7

DEDICATED
TO MY WIFE
MOLLY

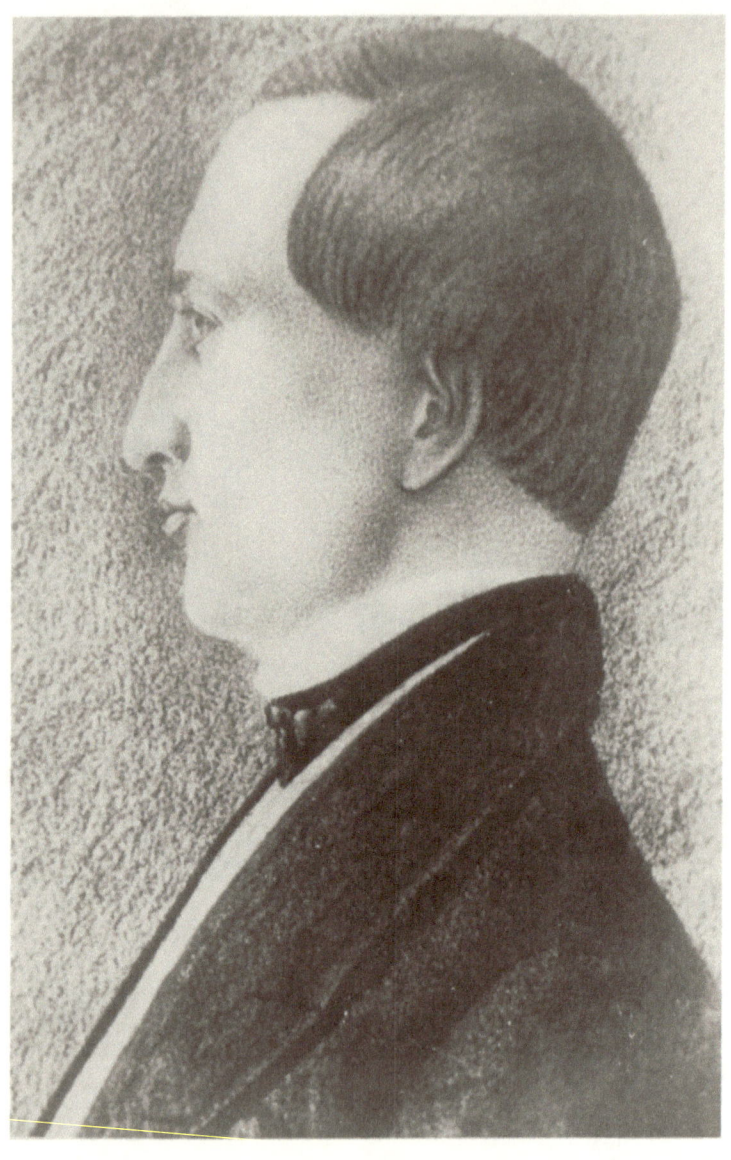

Crayon portrait of Crawford Long at the time of the first anesthetic

FOREWORD

Man's fight against pain, culminating in the discovery of the anesthetic properties of ether, opened a new heaven and a new earth to surgery. Human nature being what it is, it was to be expected that endless dispute regarding the discovery and the priority concerning its use would arise.

This controversy has continued for a century among proponents of Long, Morton, Jackson, and Wells. From it all has come the fact that Crawford Long admittedly performed the first operation with ether as the anesthetic agent, and made no effort to conceal the nature of the drug or to establish his priority. There is no doubt that Morton, some four years later, gave the first public demonstration of the anesthetic effects of ether, but attempted to conceal his formula.

Dr. Boland has worked tirelessly for many years to establish Long's priority, and now has added another chapter to the previously-known accounts of Long's life and times. That Jackson told Morton of the anesthetic effects of ether, there is little doubt. There is no authentic proof that he secured this information during his travels in Georgia, but Dr. Boland's hypothesis is an interesting one, and in view of Jackson's ubiquitous character, is probably correct.

Dr. Boland has produced a readable and interesting story, and has added a valuable chapter to the history of the greatest contribution to medicine.

Daniel C. Elkin,
Professor of Surgery,
Emory University

ACKNOWLEDGMENTS

Many acknowledgments are due in the writing of this book, and I make them with grateful appreciation. Part of the material, especially under "Ether Controversy Retold," is original, but a large amount (for which I have tried to give full credit) necessarily had to come from other sources.

By no means is the book a complete history of the discovery of surgical anesthesia. Its name indicates that it has to do with the part played by one man, Crawford Williamson Long. The whole story, a fascinating, interminable one, has been well covered by others, particularly during the past few years, in celebration of Morton's first demonstration before a medical audience in Boston in 1846.

Of recent works which have been especially helpful to me are: *History of Surgical Anesthesia*, by Thomas E. Keys; *Man Against Pain*, by Howard Riley Raper; *Victory Over Pain*, by Victor Robinson; *Centennial of Surgical Anesthesia, an Annotated Catalogue*, by John F. Fulton and Madeline E. Stanton; and the Anesthesia Centennial Number of the *Journal of the History of Medicine*, October, 1946. I am indebted principally to four writings: *Crawford W. Long and the Discovery of Anesthesia*, by his daughter, Frances Long Taylor; *Crawford W. Long, the Distinguished Physician-Pharmacist*, by his former employee, Joseph Jacobs; the article of George H. Bunch on *Charles Thomas Jackson;* and the *U. S. Congress Reports on the Ether Discovery, 1852-1863*, lent from the library of John Farquhar Fulton. Profound obligations are expressed to Dr. Fulton for the privilege of studying this important volume.

Several libraries and individuals have given indispensable information and materials: Miss Mildred Jordan, and the A. W. Calhoun Medical Library, of Emory University;

Emory University Library; Miss Carrie T. Williams, and the Carnegie Library, of Atlanta; Miss Ella May Thornton, and the State Library of Georgia; Mrs. J. E. Hays, and the Department of Archives and History of Georgia; Miss Ruth Blair, and the Atlanta Historical Society; Georgia Historical Society; and the Library and Alumni Society, University of Georgia. The original documents confirming Crawford Long's accomplishment are deposited with the Library of Congress, and we are fortunate in being able to reproduce them.

Of much value also have been letters, suggestions, and other aid from Charles C. Thomas, Springfield, Illinois; William Cole Jones, Associate Editor, *Atlanta Journal;* Charlton Ogburn, New York City; Chauncey D. Leake, University of Texas; Ralph H. Major, University of Kansas; Arno B. Luckhardt, University of Chicago; Thomas W. Reed, University of Georgia; T. B. Rice, Greensboro, Georgia; and George Ward Boland, Boston.

Also I acknowledge my debt to Miss Frances Smith, Jefferson, Georgia, for important information about Jefferson and its people; and to a member of the Long family, Mrs. James V. Webb, Athens, for procuring papers and pictures from the collection of Edward Crawford Long, grandson of Dr. Long. I thank Miss Bertha Trott, Baltimore, secretary to Dr. Hugh H. Young, for valuable photographs and literature belonging to Dr. Young, and Mrs. Logan Clendening, San Marino, California, for a copy of Crawford Long's revealing letter.

Mrs. Marion S. Harper, Atlanta, proved co-operative and capable in assembling the facts collected in reference to Georgiana Bird Washburn and her family. In this investigation Mrs. Harper was assisted by Mrs. W. W. Norman, Griffin, Georgia, a descendent of the McCleskey family; Mrs. W. R. Dancy, Savannah, Georgia in quoting old library records; Miss Rossie Wade, Milledgeville, Georgia, in quoting Bible records; Elizabeth McElhannon, Gainesville, Georgia; and Mrs. Caroline North George, Tangipahoa, Louisiana. The list of those who have helped me would not be complete without including Miss "Peggy" Nicolassen, my faithful and efficient secretary.

Appreciation and thanks are given Dr. Daniel C. Elkin, *Joseph B. Whitehead* Professor of Surgery, Emory University School of Medicine, and Dr. Isaac Starr, *Dean,* University of Pennsylvania School of Medicine, for their Statements.

Atlanta F. K. B.

CONTENTS

Foreword	v
List of Illustrations	xiii
I. PREVIOUS ATTEMPTS	3
Mesmerism	11
II. SURGERY WITHOUT ANESTHESIA	15
III. PREPARATION	21
IV. ACHIEVEMENT	31
V. COMMENT	51
The Wilhite Incident	55
VI. MORE PROOFS	59
VII. ETHER CONTROVERSY RETOLD	77
Wells	79
Morton	81
Jackson	85
"Jackson Knew How To Save A Secret"	86
Jackson Visits The Mines	88
Jackson's Account Of His Visit To Long	94
Jackson From Long	103
Jackson Knew It Would Work	108
Jackson To Morton	110
VIII. AFTERWARDS	115
Recognition	120
Conclusion	129
Appendix	133
References	145
Bibliography	151

ILLUSTRATIONS

Crayon portrait of Crawford Long at the time of
the first anesthetic ———————————————— frontispiece
FOLLOWING PAGE 36
Birthplace of Crawford Long, Danielsville, Georgia
University of Georgia at the time Long was a student
Medical Hall which was occupied by the University of Pennsylvania from 1829 until the University was moved to its present site in 1872
Mulberry tree under which stood Long's office where the first anesthetic was administered
Artist's conception of the first anesthetic, March 30, 1842
Home built and occupied by Dr. Long and his family in Atlanta, 1850
Home of Crawford Long in Athens at the time of his death
Medallion at the University of Pennsylvania. Presented in 1912
Statue of Crawford Long in Danielsville, Georgia, replica of statue in Statuary Hall, Washington, D. C.
Copy of Mrs. Frances Long Taylor's letter certifying the genuiness of her father's letter
Part of a letter in Dr. Long's handwriting to Dr. McCleskey
FOLLOWING PAGE 84
Charles T. Jackson (1805-1880)
William H. Morton (1819-1868)
Crawford Long painted by Lewis Gregg, in Alumni Hall, The University of Georgia
Eastern Massachusetts in 1841, showing relative locations of Plymouth, Bridgewater, and Boston
John C. Warren (1778-1856)
George Hayward (1791-1863)
Chair in which Jackson claimed to have discovered anesthesia, "February 1842"
Horace Wells (1815-1848)
Crawford Long Memorial Hospital, Atlanta

It has been said that surgical anesthesia is the greatest discovery of man. While it is not difficult to describe the limitless triumphs of electricity and of other marvellous inventions and discoveries, on land and sea, and in the air, which some may regard as the first in importance, to the individual who has experienced the power of surgical anesthesia to prevent pain, restore health and save life, all other human contributions become secondary in comparison. How was it found? With a towel, a bottle of ether, a prepared mind, a courageous heart, and a prayer—seemingly so simple, but creating for the world such a sublime, revolutionary gift! That was THE FIRST ANESTHETIC.

1

PREVIOUS ATTEMPTS

IT IS NOTEWORTHY THAT ALthough books and poems were written in previous centuries recommending various drugs and methods to relieve pain and cause sedation and sleep, very few agents were ever actually employed to prevent the suffering attending surgical operations. If means were used for this purpose very little is said about them in literature. Meager was the history of the early attempts at anesthesia, even up to the day when successful anesthesia was introduced. Formerly medicine was taught by didactic lectures; there was but little presentation of cases. The so-called anesthesia of our ancestors apparently followed a similar course: The subject seemed to be more philosophical and poetical than practical. In the meantime patients submitting to operative procedures underwent indescribable agonies.

Fortunately operations were few and far between as compared with modern times, and only such surgery was undertaken as could be performed with the utmost rapidity. Cutting for bladder stone probably required the longest time, often as much as half an hour, but amputations of large parts were completed in a minute or two. It seems that the forefathers in surgery felt that the use of agents to relieve pain was a confession of weakness on the part of the operator. In all his work Hippocrates, the Father of Medicine, did not deign to mention avoidance of operative tortures, while Galen, a few centuries later, declared that he abhorred drugs to alleviate pain.

Helenium was one of the first soporific drugs described. Homer said it had its origin in the tears of Helen and was to be taken in wine. Though considered a mythological concoction, fit subject for poetry only, such a drug may have existed; for, as Emerson says, myths and legends were once history. It has probably always been known that wine and later, stronger alcoholic drinks, may be responsible for varying degrees of narcosis, but were not to be depended upon for anesthesia.

As an anesthetic, mandragora (mandrake, podophillin) probably has been written about more than any other of the drugs of early days. Shakespeare has Cleopatra exclaim, "Give me to drink mandragora that I might sleep out this great gap of time my Anthony is away." Pliny the Elder, who perished in the destruction of Herculaneum, in A.D. 79, in describing the plant mandragora, says, "It has a soporific power on the faculty of those who drink it; the ordinary potion is half a cup. It is drank against serpents, and before cutting and puncturing, lest they should be felt." It was the most widely used narcotic drug, said to be the ancient equivalent of modern belladonna, the sedative effects of which are not recognized today. From all accounts, however, the older drug must have been more potent as a soporific; but Dioscorides, who recommended it for anesthesia, does not report a single case in which it was actually employed. This celebrated physician of the first century A.D. served for a time in the army of Nero and was the first to use the word

Previous Attempts

"anesthesia" when he wrote: "And some boil down in wine the roots into a third and having strained out they store away; using one cyathus upon those being sleepless and those in great pain and upon whom they wish to produce *anesthesia* while being cut or cauterized."[1] Oliver Wendell Holmes added "anesthetic"; "anesthetist" evolved later. Quistorp, of Rostock, Mecklenberg, was the author of *De Anesthesia*, published in 1718, in which he resurrected the word and used it in discussing whether the body leaves the soul when consciousness is lost under anesthesia. There is a long section in the book on why pain is not always experienced during torture, and especially during the agony of crucifixion.[2]

The *U. S. Congress Reports on the Ether Discovery*, 1863,[3] gives interesting facts concerning the first attempts in anesthesia, which are reproduced here. Hoatho, in China, about 220 A.D., is credited with the following passage: "But if the disease resided in parts upon which the needle or liquid medicaments could not operate—for example in the bones, in the stomach or intestines, he gave the patient a preparation of hemp (in Chinese, *ma-yo*,) and after a few moments he became as insensible as if he had been drunk or dead. Then, as the case required, he performed operations, incisions, or amputations, and removed the cause of the malady; then he brought together and secured the tissues, and applied liniments. After a certain number of days the patient recovered, without having experienced, during the operation, the slightest pain." This has some elements of the description of a modern operation. Hemp was also known as hashish, or *Cannabis indica*, and in more recent years has become "marijuana" in Mexico, Central and South America, but is not rated as an anesthetic drug. From the statement of Hoatho, one is led to believe that early attempts at anesthesia sometimes succeeded, after all, but the final result is rarely mentioned.

In medieval times several hypnotic sponges were introduced, the fumes from which were to be inhaled during operation, but as usual no cases are recorded to indicate the success or failure of the method. In the thirteenth century Hugh (Ugo) of Lucca, the leading surgeon of the day, and author of the principal book, *Cyrurgia*, concocted a palliative sponge described as follows by Hugh's son, Theodoric, Bishop of Cervia (1205-1298): "Take of opium, of the juice of unripe mulberry, of hyoscyamus, of the juice of hemlock, of the juice of the leaves of mandragora, of the juice of the wood-ivy, of the juice of the forest mulberry, of the seeds of lettuce, of the seeds of the dock, which has large round apples, and of the water hemlock—each an ounce, mix all these in a brazen vessel, and then place in it a new sponge; let the whole boil as long as the sun lasts on the dog-days, until the sponge consumes it all, and it is boiled away in it. As often as there shall be need of it, place this sponge in hot water for an hour, and let it be applied to the nostril of him who is to be operated upon, until he has fallen asleep, and so let the surgery be performed. This being finished, in order to awaken him, apply another sponge, dipped in vinegar, frequently to the nose, or throw the juice of the root of fenugreek into the nostrils; shortly he awakes."[4]

His father's sponge seemed effective, but Theodoric doubted its power to produce anesthesia; so he continued to bind his surgical patients. Guy de Chauliac, whose text-book ranked first in the later Middle Ages, continued to urge the use of the inhalation of narcotics. J. Canape, physician to Francis I, wrote a book in which he speaks of the procedure of Theodoric and others, and refers to the dangers of the internal administration of narcotics. The sponge of Hugh of Lucca contained about every drug that was used as a hypnotic in those days, a veritable "shotgun" prescription. Ambroise Pare, of the sixteenth century, accounted one of the greatest surgeons, stated that "a decoction of mandragora was *formerly* used to avert the pain attendant upon the amputation of a limb," but does not explain what he employed for the purpose. John Ardene, of Newark-on-Trent, originated an ointment consisting of about the same ingredients as the sponge of Hugo of Lucca. The sponge often made the patient sleep too profoundly. To prevent this, Ardene said: "And know that it is well to tweak the nose, to pinch the cheeks, or to pluck the beard of such a sleeper to quicken his spirits lest he sleep too deeply."[5]

A plausible explanation for the lack of improvement in the composition of soporific drugs during these "dark ages" was that the active principle (alkaloids) of drugs was unknown, and therefore only drugs in their primitive state were available. Better results would have been achieved if morphine, instead of crude opium, could have been used. Nevertheless, some form of opium (called by Van Helmont the "specific gift" of the Creator), before the discovery of successful inhalation anesthesia, "was the longest time in vogue, and with by far the most certain and satisfactory results. Theodoric and Guy de Chauliac gave it internally, and other surgeons advocated its use. Up to the time of the discovery of etherization it was in reality the only means relied upon to deaden the anguish of an operation. It was the custom to administer a large dose, but one varied to the age of the patient, a short time previous to the commencement of the operation, which, if grave, was never begun until the effects of the drug were manifested. Although the effect was never pushed to the state of stupefaction, and consequently a great degree of pain could be felt, opium could never be looked upon as a reliable or safe agent. The uncertainty of the time or power of its action; the delirious excitement which it often occasioned instead of insensibility; its really poisonous properties, and the subsequent troubles which it made liable—all conspired to render its use as seldom as possible, and then only for extreme cases."[6] The various alkaloids of opium are today used only as adjuncts to surgical anesthesia, before operation.

During the long experimental period before ether was used, physical agents were tried as stupefacients, with some success. Avicenna (979-1037) advised snow and ice-cold water for the purpose. The same method was employed by the Russians operating during the Second World War without adequate facilities on the battle-field, when it was found that a frozen, or nearly frozen limb could be removed with a minimum of discomfort.[7] Ethyl chloride is used today to alleviate pain by freezing the part. In 1784 James Moore in London wrote a book on preventing operative pain by placing a pressure clamp on the major nerve trunks, but he also gave a grain of opium at the same time which probably played a large part in producing anesthesia. The pioneer surgical pathologist, John Hunter, amputated a leg under this type of anesthesia, and thought the pain was considerably diminished, but there is no record of his having tried the method a second time. To show that some of the early methods of anesthesia might succeed, the *U. S. Congress Reports on the Ether Discovery* contains this passage: "M. Dauriol, a French physician residing in the neighborhood of Toulouse, asserts that, in 1832, he followed the directions given by Theodoric and operated several times with success. He even reports five cases of painless operations." To record that "letheon" was not the first secret anesthetic, the same *Report* contains an account by Meisner of a secret agent given by Weiss to Augustus II, (1670-1733), King of Poland, which produced such a perfect state of anesthesia that the King's diseased foot was amputated without his feeling it. In fact the operation was performed without the royal patient's consent, and was not discovered by him until the following morning.

Many factors delayed the coming of potent anesthesia in surgery, tradition and religious opposition being two of the principal ones. Man is a creature of habit and tradition, and from these it is hard to break him. An old saying, "What was good enough for my father is good enough for me," played a part in the cruel, senseless procrastination. As the first man and woman were driven from the Garden of Eden, she was reminded, "In sorrow thou shalt bring forth children," (*Genesis* 3:16) and for a long time many literal fundamentalists believed it should remain that way. Even today occasionally a woman in labor insists that nothing be given her to allay her pain. Years ago punishment was meted out to those who attempted to relieve the suffering of childbirth. Myra E. Babcock[8] tells of a woman, in 1591, who was buried alive for seeking such relief at the birth of her two sons.

Although ether was first described in the sixteenth century by Valerius Cordus, of Germany, three hundred years passed before its anesthetic properties were recognized. Paracelsus, the eccentric genius, in the same century hinted at it when he declared, "It quiets all suffering without harm and relieves all pain." The drug was first known as "sweet vitriol," but in 1730 Frobenius of Germany named it "ether." Joseph Priestley, in England, discovered oxygen in 1771, and nitrous oxide the following year, but the anesthetic and analgesic qualities of the latter were not recognized until April 9th, 1799, by Humphry Davy, the distinguished English scientist. In 1795 Davy inhaled nitrous oxide gas which produced such sensations of giddiness and relaxation of muscles, and altogether made him feel so cheerful that he was forced to laugh, from which arose the name "laughing gas." Afterwards came his often quoted statement, the full significance of which was so slowly appreciated, "As nitrous oxide in its extensive operation appears capable of destroying pain, it may be used with advantage during surgical operations, in which no great effusion of blood takes place." The reference to blood effusion is not clear. To study further the effects of the gas on man, Davy administered it, among others, to Roget, of Thesaurus fame, and the poets Coleridge and Southey. The effects usually bore out the name of "laughing gas."

Later in life, when Humphry Davy became president of the Royal Society, he declared that he regretted the time spent on research in nitrous oxide gas. Most writers, however, agree that his experiments formed an important stepping stone toward the discovery of surgical anesthesia and today are among Davy's principal claims to fame. Davy was not a physician, but the next Englishman to experiment with a pain-killing gas was. He was Henry Hill Hickman, whose sensitive feelings were appalled by the agonies suffered by patients undergoing surgical operations. He resolved to do something to alleviate the suffering, and very nearly succeeded. He was the first to employ carbon dioxide as an anesthetic, successfully putting puppies asleep with it, so that all manner of operations could be performed upon them. Since the animals recovered after having lost consciousness, he called the anesthetic condition "suspended animation." Many young experimentors have been discouraged, or have been forced to abandon their projects by the ridicule of their elders, but the case of Hickman is one of the most pathetic in medical annals. When he attempted to bring his experiments to the attention of surgeons at home, and on the Continent, he was met with derision, a situation hard to understand when surgery was barely surviving for want of a successful method of anesthesia. Even Davy, whose attainments had made him arrogant, would not hear the brilliant young physician. Had Hickman received the cooperation to which the success of his experiments entitled him, he might have been acclaimed the discoverer of surgical anesthesia. As it was, his bitter treatment brought early death. Since such valuable preliminary work toward the discovery of anesthesia was done by Englishmen, to take place in America, it was appropriate that many tributes be paid to Hickman in this country in 1928,[9] the one hundredth anniversary of his death.

Faraday[10] and Periera[11] also made valuable contributions toward the discovery: In 1818, a pupil of Davy, Michael Faraday, noted for his experiments in electricity, wrote, "By the imprudent inspiration of ether, a gentleman was thrown into a very lethargic state, which continued with various periods of intermission for more than thirty hours; and a great depression of spirits; for many days the pulse was so lowered that fears were entertained for his life"; and under the heading "Ether," Joseph Periera observed in 1839, "The vapor of ether is inhaled in spasmodic asthma, chronic catarrh, whooping cough, and dyspepsia, and to relieve the effects caused by the accidental inhalation of chlorine gas."

MESMERISM

Mesmerism, or hypnotism, is the last method of anesthesia attempted before the advent of triumphal surgical anesthesia, and was continued by surgeons after ether narcosis became established. It apparently approached success more nearly than any system yet undertaken, but was uncertain, because not every surgeon could administer it and not every patient could be anesthetized by it. While the name comes from Frederick A. Mesmer, a graduate of the University of Vienna who introduced the procedure in 1779, he did not suggest its use to prevent pain in surgical operations. He believed that the body contained a "magnetic fluid" which he called "animal magnetism," which was capable of curing many human ills, and asserted that he could eradicate everything from stomach-ache to paralysis, and from ear-ache to blindness. It was left mainly for three British surgeons—John Elliotson, James Esdaile, and James Braid—to apply mesmerism to surgery. They reported favorable results in many cases and wrote of the method extensively between 1843 and 1846, just at the time when inhalation anesthesia was first being tried. However, before this time, as mesmerism gained in popularity, the King of France appointed a Commission to investigate its claims. Among the members of the Commission were Benjamin Franklin, Antoine Lavoisier, and Joseph-Ignace Guillotine, after whom the decapitating device was named. The Commission reported that there was no such thing as "animal magnetism," and that therefore no cures could be expected.

The fact that mesmerism and effective anesthesia appeared at about the same time is evidence that those interested in the science of surgery realized that little further advancement could be made without some means of reducing pain during operations and that they recognized the necessity of experimentation. Hardy surgeons could perform amputations and operations on external parts of the body without anesthesia, but they must have realized that occasions frequently arose when, for example, the abdominal cavity needed to be explored, and how could this be done without the relaxing effect of complete narcosis, and how could evisceration be avoided without it? Ephraim McDowell spoke of the difficult evisceration which occurred during the ovariotomy performed upon Jane Todd Crawford in 1809, without anesthesia. The profession was not convinced of the efficiency of mesmerism, but a few members, for lack of a better pain-killer, adopted it enthusiastically for a score of years, when it died a natural death.

2

SURGERY WITHOUT ANESTHESIA

Even today, with our perfected methods of anesthesia and surgical technique, surgeons occasionally meet patients and their families who shrink from hospitals and surgical procedures, and often it is with difficulty that they can be convinced of the safety and painlessness of the necessary surgical treatment. Such fear of surgery is a survival of the old stories from the days of surgery without anesthesia and without asepsis. No one living today can picture a surgical operation without anesthesia! It was too ghastly and heart-rending. If soporific drugs were used, they had but little effect so far as pain relief was concerned. A full-blooded individual might be bled in an effort toward leading him to unconsciousness.[12] If he had not fainted, as patients sometimes did, probably would be praying that the operation be hurriedly finished or even stopped. He would implore and threaten and might escape if not firmly secured. But the operator could not faint and must finish what he had set out to do. Charles Darwin decided not to be a doctor because of these spectacles. It is inconceivable to us in our enlightened age that men as surgeons of the past whose names have been handed down with reverence could be capable of operating under these circumstances! Is it any wonder that they were called "mister" rather than "doctor"?

A historical case of amputation without anesthesia was described by John Ashhurst, Jr., in 1896, in a paper read at the fiftieth anniversary of Morton's demonstration of anesthesia at the Massachusetts General Hospital: "No braver or more gallant gentleman ever lived than Admiral Nelson. After his right elbow had been shattered by a French bullet in the assault at Teneriffe in 1797, he manifested the utmost courage, refusing to be taken to the nearest ship lest the sight of his injury should alarm the wife of a fellow-officer, whose own fate was uncertain; and when his own ship was reached, climbing up its side without assistance, and saying, 'Tell the surgeon to make haste and get his instruments. I know I must lose my right arm, so the sooner it is off the better.' He underwent the amputation, we learn from a private letter of one of his midshipmen, with the same firmness and courage that have always marked his character; and yet so painfully was he affected by the coldness of the operator's knife, that though, when next going into action at the famous battle of the Nile, he could, after calmly finishing his meal, say to his officers, 'By this time tomorrow I shall have gained a peerage or Westminster Abbey,' yet he gave standing orders to his surgeons that hot water should always be kept in readiness during an engagement, so that if another operation should be required, he might at least have the poor comfort of being cut with *warm* instruments."

A London hospital had a large bell. It was used to call all nurses and doctors not otherwise engaged to rush in and assist in holding a patient about to be submitted to operation. Before the general use of artificial lighting, operating rooms were usually placed on the top floor so that the skylight could be used to best advantage. But in some hospitals it was said that the operating room was located as high as possible not because of lighting difficulties but so that the yells and imprecations of patients undergoing operative surgery could not reach the ears of the rest of the occupants of the institution.

In the *Principles and Practice of Modern Surgery* written as late as 1847 by Robert Druitt, of England, the only reference to the care of the patient during operation is, "there should be a sufficient number of assistants to restrain the patient's struggles, to administer cordials, and a bed or table with pillows or cushions to make the patient's position as easy as possible." And further, "the operator should always cut the skin as speedily as possible, for it is the most painful part of every operation."

And these surgeons had speed. Sir Clifford Allbutt (1837-1925) wrote, "When I was a boy, surgeons operating on the quick were pitted one against the other like runners on time. He was the best surgeon, both for patient and onlooker, who broke the three minute record in an amputation or lithotomy."[13] Baron Dominique Jean Larrey, Napoleon's famous surgeon, was known to perform a shoulder-joint disarticulation in one minute, and the leading surgeons of that day were equally rapid in their manipulations. Robert Liston (1794-1847), one of the best-known Scottish surgeons of the first half of the nineteenth century, was noted for operative speed and dexterity, and he advised his associates to make rapid skin incisions and become ambidextrous. In the American editions of his text-books, although he was a forceful writer, he says very little about caring for the patient during the operation and nothing about avoiding pain. John Collins Warren[14] was a more deliberate surgeon. Observing a visiting doctor pull out his watch just as he was about to start an operation, he remarked, "You may put up your watch; I do not operate by time."

Many factors limited the number of surgical operations performed in those days. Lack of successful anesthesia and measures to prevent infections barred the study of living pathology so that the profession could not know of the great fields of human disease which could be relieved by surgical treatment. As an example, consider appendicitis. Today laymen ask what was done about this disease before it was learned that it could be cured by operating. The present writer does not think appendicitis was as frequent one hundred years ago as it is today, because of difference in *diet* in the two periods; but undoubtedly the disease did exist, as did other affections of the digestive system which now are amenable to surgery. Therefore operative pain delayed the knowledge of pathological conditions in the abdomen, and without this knowledge surgeons could not advise laparotomy. Even had surgeons been reasonably sure what was going on in the abdomen, the dread of pain would have deterred patients from submitting to operation; and so people continued to die from undiagnosed abdominal lesions. When operating was done, as Trent[15] writes: "For all patients the experience entailed severe nervous shock and a long period of depression to follow, conditions which interfered seriously with the healing of operative wounds, and greatly protracted convalescence."

Expressions like "It takes nerve and a steady hand to be a surgeon" originated in pre-anesthetic days, when there was truth in such a declaration. Operating without anesthesia, with a struggling, groaning, or yelling patient as a subject, even if one were absolutely sure of his anatomy, he must be extremely careful lest his hand might "slip," and cut something which did not require surgery. The often-quoted sentence from the American surgeon, Valentine Mott, indicates the difficulties under which the surgeon of preanesthetic operations labored: "How often, when operating

Surgery Without Anesthesia

in some deep, dark wound, along the course of some great vein, with thin walls, alternately distended and flaccid with the vital current—how often have I dreaded that some unfortunate struggle of the patient would deviate the knife a little from its normal course, and that I, who fain would be the deliverer, should involuntarily become the executioner, seeing my patient perish in my hands by one of the most appalling forms of death."[16]

Thus, while we commiserate with the unfortunate patient who was compelled to undergo the agony and shock of surgery without anesthesia, we must not forget the terrible ordeal of the surgeon. Nothing must overcome his coolness and presence of mind. His manual dexterity had to excel that of surgeons of today, *and it did.* As has been charged, probably some surgeons became "hardened" by their harrowing experiences, a reaction which erroneously has been supposed to exist sometimes today. Verily, anesthesia has been a potent factor in increasing man's average longevity from thirty-five years at the time of the War Between the States to sixty-seven years today, both among patients and among doctors!

Luckily, and necessarily, operations before the introduction of anesthesia were few, and were attempted only as a last resort. Robinson[17] states that during the five years immediately preceding anesthesia only 184 operations, about three a month, were performed at the Massachusetts General Hospital, a surprising total for such a large institution. These were confined chiefly to the surface of the body, including excision of tumors, amputation of limbs and breasts, ligations, plastic operations, herniotomies and lithotomies. *The number of operations trebled during the five years following the introduction of anesthesia.* In 1844-45, Liston's operative list was as follows: lithotomy, 5 cases; herniotomy, 4; tumors excised, 22 including a large ovarian tumor; amputations, 10; excision of joint, 1; ligation of aneurism, 1; perineal section for lacerated urethra, 1; operations for phimosis and fistula in-ano, and several plastics. Liston was one of the leading surgeons of the world at this time, but this was enough surgery without anesthesia.

About the only other operations performed over the world during the first half of the nineteenth century were trephining, probably the oldest of all, as shown in prehistoric skulls; thoracotomy, which was done by Hippocrates; and the reductions of fractures and dislocations. Except in a few instances, like McDowell's, the abdomen was invaded only in extensive trauma. Without anesthesia, such a thing as an exploratory laparotomy was unthinkable. Most of the operations which have been mentioned were performed in ancient times as well as in the nineteenth century, so that it is seen that because of the lack of effective anesthesia, surgery had made but little progress in thousands of years. As the advent of anesthesia drew nearer, surgeons were becoming bolder, and operating more frequently, thus increasing the demand for means to prevent pain.

A significant factor in postponing the introduction of successful surgical anesthesia was the lack of knowledge of the possibilities of operative surgical treatment. Such knowledge gradually began to dawn after anesthesia became established. Formerly, operating without anesthesia seemed satisfactory enough for amputations and the other operations of the day; the profession and the public had become so long accustomed to it. Had it been recognized that the great cavities of the body could be safely invaded with the patient asleep and relaxed, more strenuous efforts would probably have been put forth to discover a satisfactory anesthetic, and such a discovery might have been made at an earlier date.

3

PREPARATION

THE SAYING OF PASTEUR THAT "In the realm of observation chance only favors the mind prepared" has but few exceptions. The life of Crawford Williamson Long, the first surgical anesthetist, proved no exception. The preparation for his epochal discovery began with his ancestry and continued with his training. His paternal grandfather, Samuel Long, was born in the province of Ulster, Ireland, and there married Ann Williamson. On the same ship with his two brothers, James and Andrew, Samuel sailed for America, and settled in the Cumberland Valley, near Carlisle, Pennsylvania, where many Scotch-Irish Presbyterians had located in 1739. The date of the arrival is not given by Mrs. Frances Long Taylor[18] in the sketch of her father, Dr. Long, but it was 1761.* She quotes from a letter written by a descendent of Samuel Long's brother who remained in Ireland:

"It is well known that the Longs were at the defense of Londonderry. They took an active and fearless part in the

---

* The dates 1739 and 1761 were furnished the writer by the Virginia Historical Society.

daring deeds of bravery of the siege, from the closing of the gates on the 18th of December, 1688, by the thirteen apprentice boys of Derry in the face of King James' Army, until they were opened on the following twelfth of August, 1689. Henry Long was Mayor of Londonderry shortly after the siege. For political reasons the Longs, with others, were dispossessed of their lands, the King giving them to his favorites along with titles of nobility. These newly made lords were generally absentees who spent their time in London and on the Continent. As the years passed the Longs became once more very prosperous, as did many others in the province of Ulster. The agent of the absentee lord called to collect the rent. 'On hospitable thoughts intent' a fine dinner was served to which he was invited. At the close of the dinner he arose and said: 'You seem to be prosperous in every way and you can afford to have silver on your table (which was rare in those days) and your rent will be increased'."

The increase was not met, and the brothers soon came to America where all three fought in the war for independence from the mother country. In 1788 Samuel Long settled in Madison County, Georgia, where he is buried in the yard of Old New Hope, the Presbyterian church which he helped to found. His son, James, father of Crawford Long, had been born in Carlisle, Pennsylvania, in 1781, and had also moved to Madison County, Georgia, the county seat of which was Danielsville. James Long was studious, fond of reading, and he received the best advantages the country then afforded. He inherited some money and Negroes from his father, and while yet a young man, by his industry and thrift had accumulated a fortune, which was to be a great help to the future young physician. James Long owned the first store in Danielsville, and was the town's first postmaster, and for years was clerk of the court. He established the first flour

Preparation 23

mill in that part of the state, and became a large stockholder in the Georgia Railroad, one of the earliest to be built in the South. He founded the Danielsville Academy and represented his district in the state Senate. He was prominent in church affairs, dignified and cultured, as became a Presbyterian elder, and altogether was recognized as a leading citizen of the state. His closest friend was William H. Crawford, of Georgia, secretary of war, minister to France, and candidate for President of the United States defeated by John Quincy Adams. James Long named his first child Crawford in honor of this friend and contemporary. Crawford Long's mother was beautiful Elizabeth Ware, a Virginia woman of Scotch-Irish ancestry, whose superior character was an influential factor in the development of her son. Her maternal grandfather was Solomon Strickland, Sr., who was born in Ireland in 1735, and located in Madison County, Georgia, where in 1756 he married Amy Pace. Their eleventh child, Jane, married Captain Edward Ware, whose daughter was Elizabeth. Both Solomon Strickland and Edward Ware fought in the Revolutionary War; so Crawford Long was a true son of the American Revolution. The Strickland family became prominent in several states of the South.*

Crawford Long was born in Danielsville, November 1, 1815, in the home to which his mother went as a bride. The house is still standing and may best be identified by its fine oak paneling, unusual in that community, which is described as being an original part of the structure. Crawford was a quiet, studious, normal boy, loving horses, dogs, swimming and fishing, and taking part in athletic sports. He entered Franklin College,** at Athens, the predecessor of the Uni-

---

* Mrs. Marion S. Harper supplied the data about the Strickland family.
** Benjamin Franklin once represented colonial Georgia in London. See E. M. Coulter: *College Life in the Old South*. The Macmillian Company, New York, 1928, p. 17.

versity of Georgia, at fourteen years of age, and graduated in 1835 with an A.M. degree, and *second honor*. It is said he would have taken first honor except for the fact that he refused to testify against a fellow student who was charged with some minor offense. It is interesting that Long's roommate in the old college building on the campus, known as "Yahoo," was Alexander H. Stephens, governor of Georgia and vice-president of the Confederacy, and one of the state's most famous men.

Throughout all his training Crawford Long was associated with successful, distinguished men. Among his contemporaries at Franklin College was Howell Cobb, who later became governor, speaker of the United States House of Representatives and senator. Cobb was secretary of the treasury during President Buchanan's administration, and was a general in the Confederate Army. Long also was associated with A. O. Bacon and Herschel Johnson, who rose to be leading United States Senators; Benjamin M. Palmer, who became a noted Presbyterian divine; Joseph and John LeConte, eminent scientists, who later were members of the faculty of the University of California; and Henry L. Benning, and Francis Bartow, who became Confederate generals. The embryo physician must have received inspiration from association with men of this mold. The college faculty of the period, while small, consisted of able teachers, headed by Alonzo Church.

Following his graduation in Athens, Long remained for one year at his home in Danielsville. His father thought nineteen too young for one to begin the study of medicine. During this interval Crawford was principal of the local academy. He had decided to become a doctor, and "read" medicine under Dr. George R. Grant of Jefferson, Georgia. It was customary in those days, and for many years later, for a prospective medical student to "read" medicine by studying the books in some practitioner's office and helping him occasionally with his patients. Often this was the sum of the medical education ever received; the young man did not matriculate with any school, and ultimately grew a practice of his own. Manifestly this was before the era of medical examining boards. In increasing numbers, however, more such students did graduate as physicians, although the preliminary "reading" of medicine for a year or two under an experienced competent physician was not time wasted.

Several theories have been advanced as to why Crawford Long first matriculated with the Medical Department of Transylvania University at Lexington, Kentucky, in 1836, and in 1838 transferred to the University of Pennsylvania. These were two of the oldest medical schools in the country, and both were justly famous. Founded in 1799, in "an outpost of civilization."* the Transylvania school, in 1836, registered the remarkable attendance of 262 medical students,[19] comparing favorably with the enrollment of any American institution of the times. Its faculty included several distinguished men, among them Benjamin Winslow Dudley, one of the world's greatest lithotomists. He was professor of surgery and it was reported that he did not lose a single patient from whom he removed a stone in the bladder, in his first one hundred cases, and only three in the 255 subsequently on his list. He was an alumnus of the Pennsylvania school, as were Caldwell, Short and Mitchell, and perhaps other teachers. With more than 10,000 books, some ancient and rare, gathered from all over the world, the Transylvania Medical Library** still remains a marvel of its kind.

* Elkin, Dan Collier: The Transylvania School and Oliver Perry Hill. *Annals of Medical History*, V-4, Paul B. Hoeber, Inc., New York, 1923, pp. 387-393.
** Charles A. Vance, "The Transylvania Medical Library," President's Address. *Transactions of the Southern Surgical Association*, LVII, J. B. Lippincott Co., 1945, pp. 1-29.

Apparently the school had reached the peak of its remarkable success at the time Crawford Long became a student. However, the next year, 1837, a serious disruption occurred when Charles Caldwell, one of the ablest and most colorful professors, was expelled from the faculty when it was discovered that he was taking part in the establishment of another medical school in Louisville. Probably for this reason, and for others, the star of the Transylvania Medical Department now began to decline, so that in 1857 the institution was discontinued. These changes in the school may have influenced Long in his decision to transfer to the Medical School of the University of Pennsylvania, or he may have been affected by the difficulties of travel to Lexington, or perhaps he was drawn to Pennsylvania because his American ancestors had first settled in that state.

His trip to Lexington, in 1836, on horseback, was long and fatiguing, and not without danger, since the Cherokees had not all been removed from western North Carolina and eastern Tennessee. After several weeks of climbing mountains, fording streams and following trails through the forests, he reached the fertile fields and blue-grass region of Kentucky. In Lexington he visited the hospitable home of Henry Clay at Ashland. His father had always been an ardent supporter of Mr. Clay, and this fact may have caused the latter to treat the young Georgian with special consideration.

In 1838 Long entered the Medical School of the University of Pennsylvania, at Philadelphia, of which it was said that "nowhere else could he have found the scientific traditions and the intellectual stimulus to original thought." This institution was looked upon as first among the twenty-eight medical schools then established in the country. Philip Syng Physic, the pupil of John Hunter, called the Father of American surgery, died during Long's first course at Pennsylvania, so that it is doubtful if Long had the advantage of learning from this celebrated teacher. At the time of his death Physic was emeritus professor of surgery. He devised the stomach tube, and many useful instruments, and was the first to use catgut as a ligature material. William Gibson, the pupil of Sir Charles Bell, succeeded Physic as professor of surgery. He had served under Wellington in Belgium, and was wounded at Waterloo. His text-book on surgery was in use at Pennsylvania. Nathaniel Chapman, whose *Therapeutics* was the text-book of the day, was professor of physic and clinical medicine, and was considered one of the most capable teachers in America.

George B. Wood, the profound scholar, the keen observer and original thinker, taught materia medica. With Franklin Bache he edited the *United States Dispensatory*. For many years he practically determined the views of the whole profession on ethics and practice. His lectures were the pride and glory of the University and had immense influence in molding the minds of the students. *His condemnation of the premature reporting of drug actions undoubtedly played a part in Long's delay a few years later in publishing his experience with ether.* Wood insisted that an observer should not be content with a single experiment. William Horner, the discoverer of the tensor tarsi muscle, was professor of anatomy. Hugh L. Hodge was professor of midwifery, having defeated Charles D. Meigs for the chair. Hodge's forceps and pessaries had world-wide reputation. Robert Hare, one of the ablest chemists and electricians of the times, was professor of chemistry. His volume on chemistry and *Horner's Anatomy* were the text-books used in the school. Besides these regular teachers on the faculty, the students heard lectures and attended clinics directed by luminaries like Robley Dunglison, Joseph Pancoast, William W. Gerhard, John Rhea Barton, and others.

Such were the men composing Pennsylvania's medical

faculty under whom Crawford Long studied. An effort has been made to find one or more text-books which he used during these formative years in the hope of discovering some early interests in trying to relieve the suffering of surgical operations. His "walking the hospitals" in New York, however, where he saw more operations, may have turned his thoughts toward the possibility of anesthesia, though he did not know the word at the time. All through his life, Long, like many physicians and surgeons today, did not write as fully and as often as his training and experience had equipped him to do. His usual excuse was the old one: *lack of time.* The young physician who puts off his first attempt at authorship too long will hardly ever "get around to it." However, very few young men have had as much to write about as did Crawford Long. His contact with efficient and progressive instructors, the best the country afforded, helped prepare him for the stroke of genius which he was destined to make a few months later.

Long first learned of the exhilarating and soporific effects of nitrous oxide gas and ether while at college in Philadelphia, in 1838 and 1839. A group of Georgia medical students boarded with two Quaker maiden ladies at the corner of Market and Nineteenth streets, where the boys locked themselves in a bedroom and tried the effects of ether for the purpose of exhilaration and not from any scientific motive.

After his graduation in medicine in 1839 Long went to New York to perfect himself further, and spent eighteen months "walking the hospitals." Here he witnessed great suffering in operations without successful efforts to relieve the pain. His record for skillful surgical assistance was so satisfactory that he was advised to go into the Navy, but, yielding to his father's wishes, he decided to return to Georgia. We have no written detailed record of his experience in New York, but know that he had opportunity at that time to learn from such recognized surgeons and teachers as Valentine Mott, Kearney Rogers, and Willard Parker. If the young surgeon had remained in New York, as many Southern boys have done since, one cannot help but speculate what would have been the outcome in regard to the publication of his first anesthetic—or would there have been any publication?

When Dr. Long came back to Georgia in 1841, he located in Jefferson, which was twenty-five miles west of Danielsville and a larger place. Less than one year later, when twenty-six years of age, he gave the first surgical anesthetic. Jefferson was a town of only a few hundred people, eighteen miles from Athens, surrounded by plantations and slaves, the planters' families being about the only white people in the community. At this time the population of Georgia was 516,823, of whom 217,530 were slaves. The chief cities were Savannah, Augusta, and Milledgeville. Atlanta did not come into existence until 1837, when it was known as Terminus, and was called Atlanta ten years later. Chapin's *United States Gazeteer* of 1839 stated that "until recently a large portion of the state was occupied by the Cherokee Indians. and the Western part by the Creeks, who had been removed to the lands assigned them by the United States west of Arkansas." Augusta and Savannah each had less than 8,000 inhabitants.

With his extraordinary preparation the young physician soon acquired as extensive a practice as he could handle with existing travel difficulties. In order to reach his patients, dangerous streams had to be forded and long drives taken over rough and lonely clay roads. Nowhere was there a good road, and horseback was the constant means of transportation. At night he rode his favorite horse, Charley, which, on account of its sagacity and sure-footedness, was invaluable to him. Once called to make a visit many miles distant on a stormy-pitch-black night, as often was his custom, he gave Charley the reins. When he arrived at a bridge, it was with difficulty that the horse could be persuaded to cross it, but with slow and hesitating steps he finally did. Long spoke of this after reaching his destination and was told his horse had carried him on a narrow foot bridge, which was a makeshift substitute to be used until a new bridge could be built to replace the old one which had been torn away. Crawford Long endured all the hardships which in those times befell the lot of the country doctor.

4

ACHIEVEMENT

WHEN IT IS STATED THAT DR. Crawford W. Long administered the first anesthetic, it is understood to mean the first *surgical* anesthetic. For many years nitrous oxide gas and ether had been used for various purposes to produce partial or complete narcosis, but Long was the first to employ effective anesthesia in a surgical operation, and by a method which became permanently and universally adopted. H. M. Lyman,[20] in 1881, wrote that William E. Clarke, a chemistry student in Rochester, New York, and afterward a prominent physician of Chicago, gave ether in January, 1842, for the extraction of a tooth by a dentist, Dr. Elijah Pope. Clarke did not claim to be the discoverer of anesthesia, he furnished no proofs of it and his contribution was not mentioned in his biography.[21] He antedated Wells in dental anesthesia rather than Long in surgical anesthesia.

"Ether parties" and "laughing gas" demonstrations became popular in parts of the United States in the early years of the nineteenth century. With no radios and moving pictures the world must be entertained in some fashion.

Quilting parties, candy pullings, and square dances enlivened social gatherings. Itinerant showmen travelled about the country giving demonstrations of amazing chemical reactions, and usually concluded the performance by inviting members of the audience to inhale the wonderful agent, laughing gas, which would cause individuals to cut up ludicrous antics and fall around and down, to the amusement and satisfaction of the crowd. It is said that Samuel Colt[22] of Hartford, Connecticut, earned some of the money he needed to perfect his revolver by becoming one of these showmen. Such parties did not appear in Jefferson, Georgia, until Crawford Long arrived in 1841 to begin the practice of medicine.

Before reading Dr. Long's description of the first operation under anesthesia, it is well to reproduce a letter written by him to Robert Goodman ordering the ether. Goodman formerly lived in Jefferson, but at the time the letter was written he had moved to Athens. The letter did not come into the possession of Mrs. Taylor until October, 1905, when it was brought to her by Mr. Goodman, then a man more than eighty years old. He said that the letter had been found in an old trunk by a member of his family. It was folded to form its own envelope as was the custom in those days, sealed with wax, and unstamped but marked "postage 25 cents." The *stage* that is referred to in the letter ran a regular route from Augusta through Washington, Athens, Jefferson, and Gainesville, to Dahlonega, and it will receive further notice. The letter read as follows:

Jefferson, Feb. 1st, 1842

Dear Bob:

I am under the necessity of troubling you a little. I am entirely out of ether and wish some by tomorrow night if it is possible to receive it by that time. You will please hand the order below to Dr. Reese, and if you can meet with an opportunity to send the medicines to me tomorrow you will confer a great favor by doing so. If you cannot send them tomorrow, get Dr. Reese to send them by the stage on Wednesday.

Your friend,
C. W. Long.

On the outside appears this notation:

"This letter written to me by Dr. C. W. Long in which he ordered the ether with which he performed the first surgical operation on a patient under the influence of that drug. A wen removed from the neck of a young man, Mr. James Venable, without giving him any pain, it was a complete success. In November, 1841, Dr. C. W. Long told me he believed an operation could be performed without the patient feeling pain by giving him ether to inhale. In April, 1842 he told me his experiment on James Venable was successful. I also saw James Venable the same spring who told me he felt no pain during the operation.

R. H. Goodman."

A photostatic copy of this letter, with Goodman's comment, is reproduced in this volume, as are similar copies of other letters and affidavits. Inasmuch as Charles T. Jackson claimed that he discovered anesthesia in February, 1842, when he experienced the effects of the inhalation of ether, Goodman's quotation from Long is interesting, when he wrote that Dr. Long told him in November, 1841, that he believed a surgical operation could be performed without the patient's feeling pain by giving him ether to inhale. However, the discovery of surgical anesthesia did not rest upon a theory or a surmise, but upon an actual operation performed successfully without pain. This, Crawford Long was the first to do. He may have been, and was, timid in writing, but not in doing! In his achievement he obeyed John Hunter's axiom, "Don't think; try."

It is best to tell of the first anesthetic in the words of the anesthetist. His first written account, with which he included important documentary evidence, printed below, was published in the *Southern Medical and Surgical Journal*, December, 1849. A more detailed report was desirable, but it must be remembered that the paper was not written until more than seven years after the epochal event, and his notes were incomplete. August Schachner,[23] Ephraim McDowell's biographer, says of McDowell's famous operation on Jane Todd Crawford, in 1809: "On such occasions historians are absent; moreover, in those times notes were seldom kept by anyone, and from all accounts by McDowell, never." Even today procrastination impairs or destroys many valuable medical reports. Long's description, however, while meager in details, was clear and conclusive, and furnishes enough to tell that the operation was actually performed, and without pain. It is not said whether the patient sat in a chair, or lay on a bed or a table. The account of a later operation describes a bed as being used, while a correspondent of the present writer declares that she owns a dining-room table, seating fourteen people, upon which the first operation was performed. The excised tumor probably was a sebaceous cyst, or wen, and one observer wrote that the young man wished it removed because it was "unsightly."

From his four years of study and observation as a student and graduate in medicine, Crawford Long realized keenly the crying need of an efficient agent for the relief of the agony of surgical operations, and although he had been practicing less than a year circumstances dramatically played into his hands. Doubtless similar situations had been presented to other young doctors, but Long took advantage of the golden opportunity. His paper, including the description of the operation, is presented herewith in full:

Southern
MEDICAL AND SURGICAL JOURNAL
Vol. 5   New Series, December, 1849.   No. 12.

Original Communications.

An account of the first use of Sulphuric Ether by Inhalation as an Anaesthetic in Surgical Operations. By C. W. Long, M.D., of Jefferson, Jackson Co., Georgia.

For nearly three years, the various medical journals have contained numerous articles on the employment of Sulphuric Ether by Inhalation for the purpose of rendering patients insensible to pain during surgical operations.

The first notice I saw of the use of ether, or rather of Dr. Morton's "Letheon," as an anaesthetic, was in the editorial of the *Medical Examiner* for December, 1846, in which the editor gives the following extract from a paper by Dr. H. J. Bigelow, contained in the *Boston Journal*: "The preparation (letheon) is inhaled from a small two-necked glass globe, and smells of ether, and is, we have little doubt, an ethereal solution of some narcotic substance."

Having on several occasions used ether, since March, 1842, to prevent pain in surgical operations, immediately after reading this notice of "letheon," I commenced a communication to the editor of the *Medical Examiner*, for publication in that Journal, to notify the medical profession that sulphuric ether, would of itself render surgical operations painless, and that it had been used by me for that purpose for more than four years. I was interrupted when I had written but a few lines, and was prevented, by a very laborious country practice, from resuming my communication, until the *Medical Examiner* for January, 1847, was received, which reached me in a few days after reading the December number. It contained several articles, giving accounts of different experiments in etherization, in which surgical operations were performed without pain. On reading these articles I determined to wait a few months before publishing an account of my discovery, and see whether any surgeon would present a claim to having used ether by inhalation in surgical operations prior to the time it was used by me.

A controversy soon ensued between Messrs. Jackson, Morton and Wells, in regard to who was entitled to the honor of being the discoverer of the anaesthetic powers of ether, and a considerable time elapsed before I was able to ascertain the exact period when their first operations were performed. Ascertaining this fact, through negligence I have now permitted a much longer time to elapse than I designed, or than my professional friends with whom I consulted advised; but as no account has been published (so far as I have been able to ascertain) of the inhalation of ether being used to prevent pain in surgical operations as early as March, 1842, my friends think I would be doing myself injustice, not to notify my brethren of the medical profession of my priority of the use of ether by inhalation in surgical practice.

I know that my interests have suffered from not making an earlier publication, and I would not be persuaded at this late stage of the ether controversy to present my claim to being the first to use ether as an anaesthetic in surgical operations, if I were not fully satisfied of my ability to establish its justice.

In the month of December, 1841, or January, 1842, the subject of the inhalation of nitrous oxide gas was introduced in a company of young men assembled at night in this village (Jefferson) and several persons present desired me to prepare some for their use. I informed them I had no apparatus for preparing or preserving the gas, but I had a medicine (sulphuric ether) which would produce equally exhilarating effects; that I had inhaled it myself, and considered it as safe as the nitrous oxide gas. One of the company stated that he had inhaled ether while at school, and was then willing

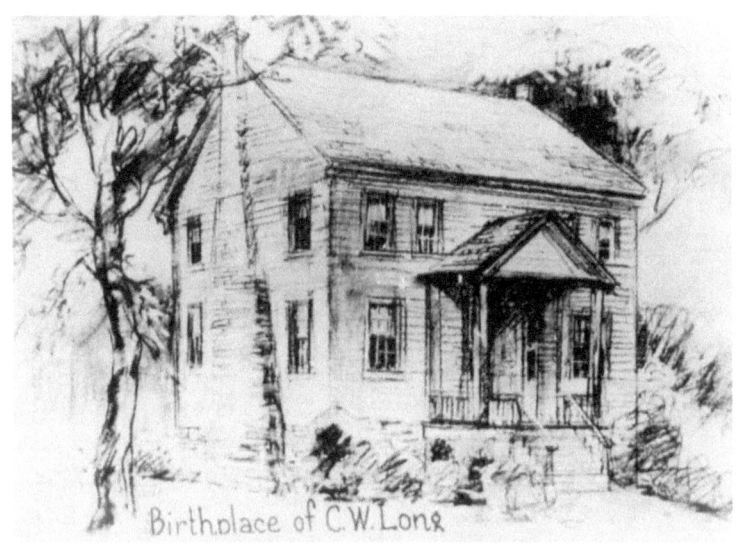

Birthplace of Crawford Long, Danielsville, Georgia
from the collection of Dr. Hugh H. Young

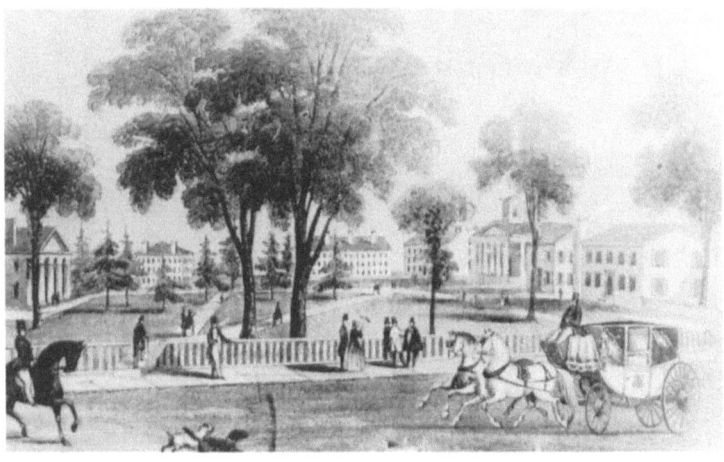

University of Georgia at the time Long was a student
University of Georgia Library

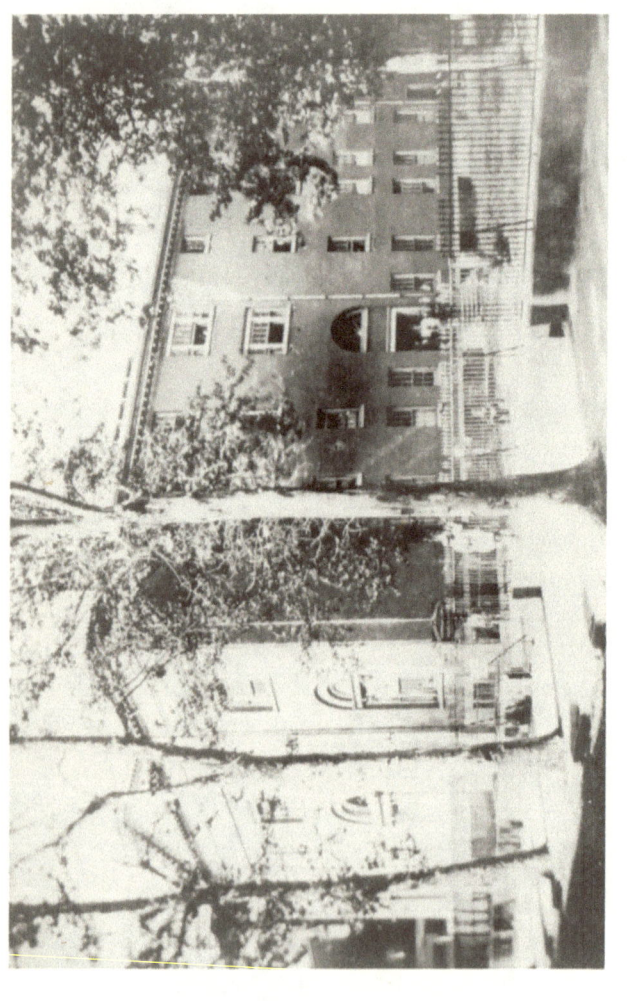

Medical Hall which was occupied by the University of Pennsylvania from 1829 until the University was moved to its present site in 1872
Courtesy Dr. Isaac Stone

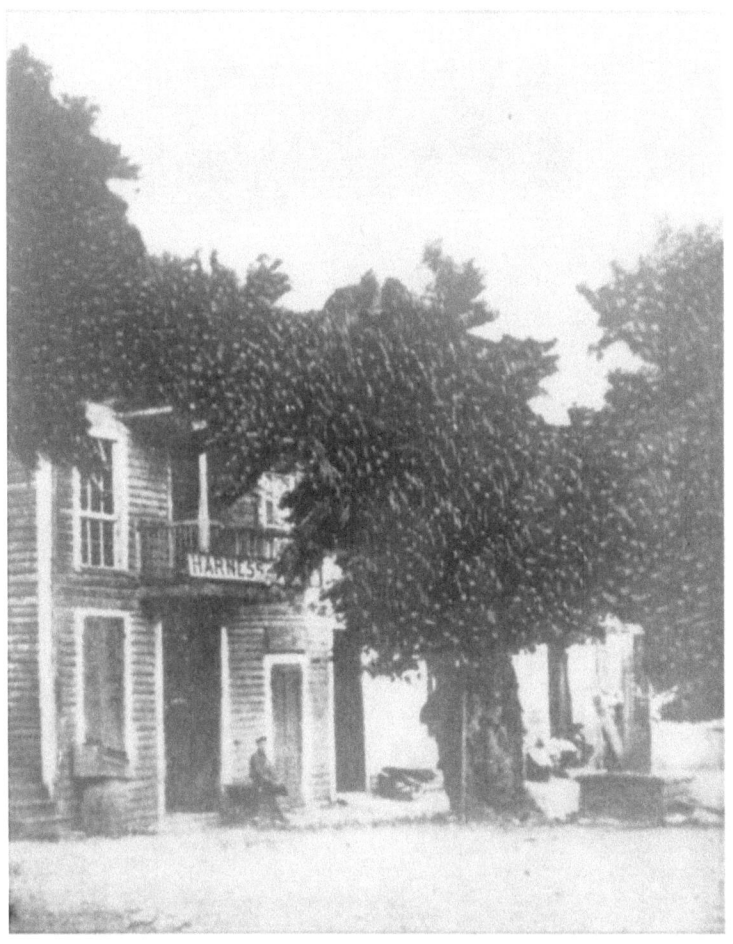

Mulberry tree under which stood Long's office where the first anesthetic was administered

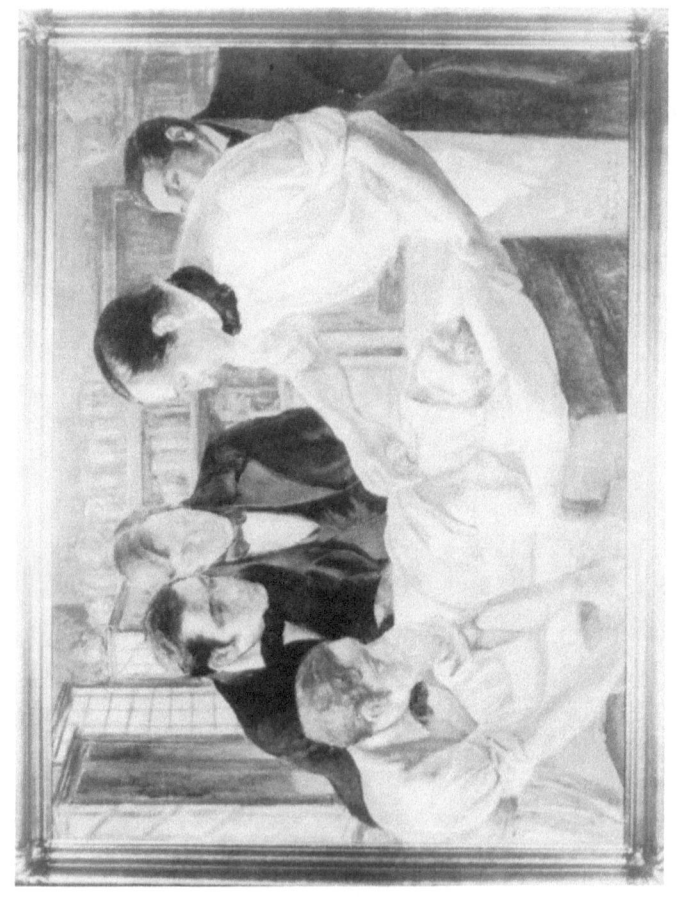

Artist's conception of the first anesthetic, March 30, 1842
Painted by Maurice Siegler

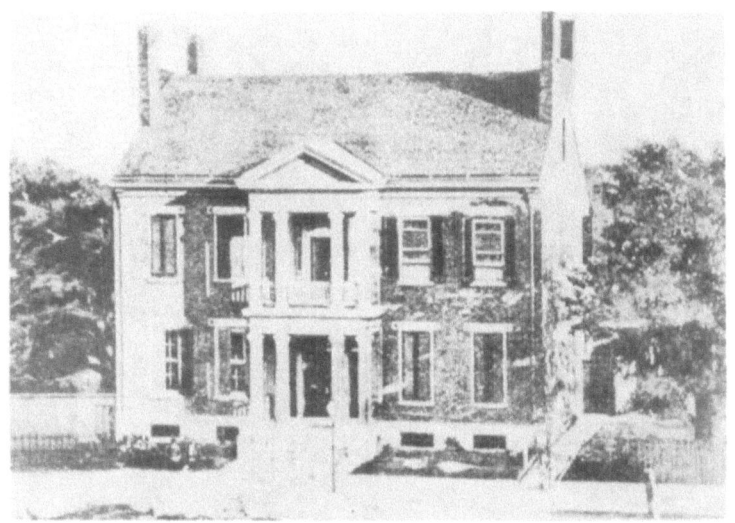

Home built and occupied by Dr. Long and his family in Atlanta, 1850

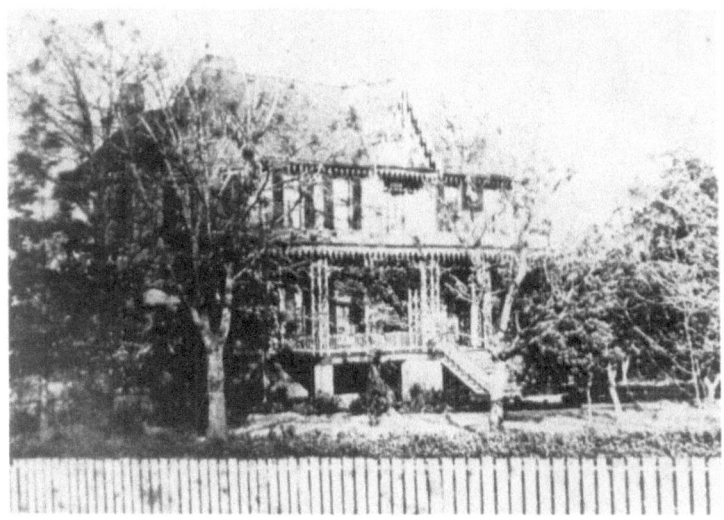

Home of Crawford Long in Athens at the time of his death.

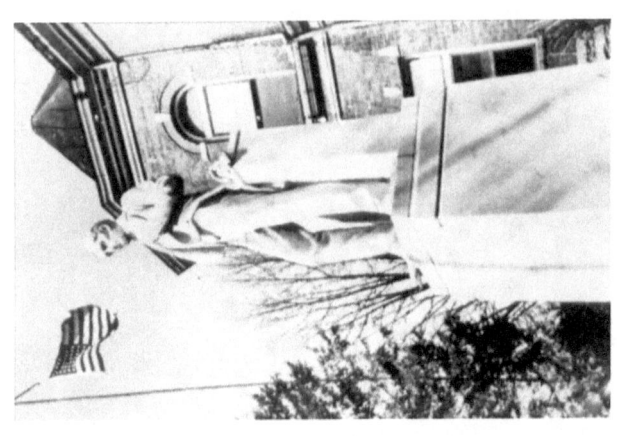

Statue of Crawford Long in Danielsville, Georgia, replica of statue in Statuary Hall, Washington, D. C.
Courtesy of The Atlanta Journal

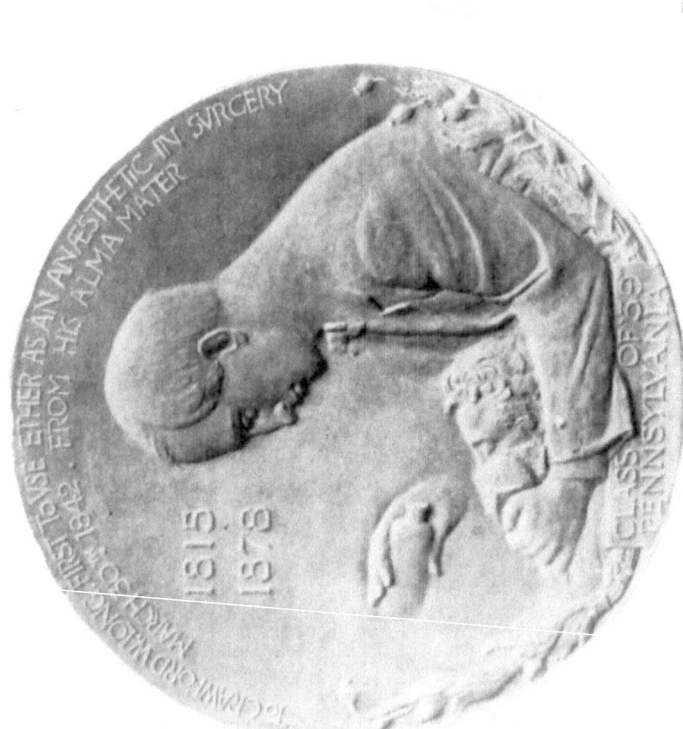

Medallion at the University of Pennsylvania. Presented in 1912

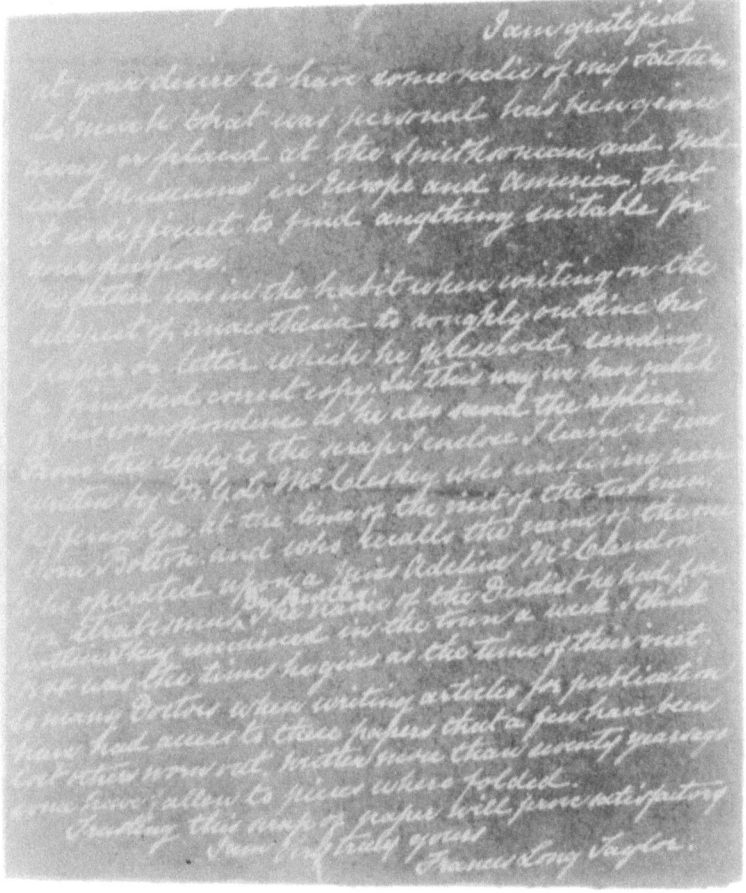

Copy of Mrs. Frances Long Taylor's letter certifying genuiness of her father's letter.
From Clendening Collection—Mrs. Logan Clendening

> *Permit me to say here that I have placed a strong belief, that Dr Wells or Morton, were in Jefferson Jackson Co. Ga in 1842 or thereing, while there was never both of my operations & obtained the knowledge of Anaesthetic products of Ether at that time — In one of these years, there was a Dentist & also operator for defects & diseases of the eye, from Boston. Their names I have been unable to ascertain &*

Part of letter written in Dr. Long's own handwriting to Dr. McCleskey, as testified by his daughter, Mrs. Frances Long Taylor. From the Long collection. An almost identical letter was found in the Clendening collection.

Part of a letter in Dr. Long's handwriting to Dr. McCleskey

From the Long collection

to inhale it. The company were all anxious to witness its effects. The ether was introduced: I gave it first to the gentleman who had previously inhaled it, then inhaled it myself, and afterwards gave it to all persons present. They were so much pleased with the exhilarating effects of ether, that they afterwards inhaled it frequently, and induced others to do so, and its inhalation soon became quite fashionable in this county, and in fact extended from this place through several counties in this part of Georgia.

On numerous occasions I have inhaled ether for its exhilarating properties, and would frequently, at some short time subsequent to its inhalation, discover bruises or painful spots on my person, which I had no recollection of causing, and which I felt satisfied were received while under the influence of ether. I noticed my friends, while etherized, received falls and blows, which I believed were sufficient to produce pain on a person not in a state of anesthesia, and on questioning them, they uniformly assured me that they did not feel the least pain from these accidents. These facts are mentioned that the reasons may be apparent why I was induced to make an experiment in etherization.

The first patient to whom I administered ether in a surgical operation was Mr. James M. Venable, who then resided within two miles of Jefferson, and at present lives in Cobb county, Georgia. Mr. Venable consulted me on several occasions in regard to the propriety of removing two small tumors situated on the back part of his neck, but would postpone from time to time having the operations performed, from dread of pain. At length I mentioned to him the fact of my receiving bruises while under the influence of the vapour of ether, without suffering, and as I knew him to be fond of, and accustomed to inhale ether, I suggested to him the probability that the operations might be performed without pain, and proposed operating upon him while under its influence. He consented to have one tumor removed, and the operation was performed the same evening.

The ether was given to Mr. Venable on a towel; and when fully under its influence I extirpated the tumour. It was encysted, and about half an inch in diameter. The patient continued to inhale ether during the time of the operation; and when informed it was over, seemed incredulous, until the tumour was shown him. He gave no evidence of suffering during the operation, and assured me, after it was over, that he did not experience the slightest degree of pain from its performance. *This operation was performed on the 30th of March, 1842.*

The second operation I performed upon a patient etherized was on the 6th of June, 1842, and was on the same person, for the removal of another small tumour. This operation required more time than the first, from the cyst of the tumour having formed adhesions to the surrounding parts. The patient was insensible to pain during the operation, until the last attachment of the cyst was separated, when he exhibited signs of slight suffering but asserted, after the operation was over, that the sensation of pain was so slight as scarcely to be perceived. In this operation the inhalation of ether ceased before the first incision was made; since that time I have invariably desired patients when practicable, to continue its inhalation during the time of the operation. Having so long neglected presenting my claim to the discovery of the anesthetic powers of ether; for the purpose of satisfying the minds of all, of its justness, I have procured, I conceive, a sufficient number of certificates to establish the claim indisputable. I present first, the certificate of James M. Venable, the patient on whom the first experiments in etherization were made, and no comments on it, I conceive, are necessary.

(Certificates.)

I, James M. Venable, of the county of Cobb and State of Georgia, on oath, depose and say, that in the year 1842, I resided at my mother's, in Jackson county, about two miles from the village of Jefferson, and attended the village

Achievement 39

academy that year. In the early part of the year the young men of Jefferson, and the country adjoining, were in the habit of inhaling ether, for its exhilarating powers, and I inhaled it myself frequently for that purpose, and was very fond of its use.

While attending the academy, I was frequently in the office of Dr. C. W. Long, and having two tumours on the side and rather back of my neck, I several times spoke to him about the propriety of cutting them out, but postponed the operation from time to time. On one occasion, we had some conversation about the probability that the tumours might be cut out while I was under the influence of s. ether, without my experiencing pain, and he proposed operating upon me while under its influence. I agreed to have one tumour cut out, and had the operation performed that evening after school was dismissed. This was in the early part of the spring of 1842.

I commenced inhaling the ether before the operation was commenced, and continued it until the operation was over. I did not feel the slightest pain from the operation, and could not believe the tumour was removed until it was shown to me.

A month or two after this time, Dr. C. W. Long cut out the other tumour, situated on the same side of my neck. In this operation I did not feel the least pain until the last cut was made, when I felt a little pain. In this operation, I stopped inhaling the ether before the operation was finished. I inhaled the ether, in both cases, from a towel, which was the common method of taking it.

James M. Venable.

GEORGIA, Cobb county,)
    July 23rd, 1849   )
        Sworn to before me
                Alfred Manes, J.P.

I certify that I was a pupil in the Academy in Jefferson,

Jackson county, in the year 1842. Some time during the spring of that year I was present, and witnessed Dr. C. W. Long cut out a small tumour from the neck of James M. Venable. I am well acquainted with the smell of sulphuric ether, and know that Mr. Venable inhaled it, before and during the time of the operation. He made no sign of suffering pain during the operation; and after the tumour was cut out, he asserted that he did not feel any pain from the cutting out of the tumour.

A few months after this operation, Mr. Venable informed me that Dr. Long had cut out another tumour from his neck, while he was under the effects of ether, and that he did not feel any pain from the operation. Mr. Venable was a pupil in the Academy during the year 1842, and I was intimate with and heard him speak of the operations frequently, and he always asserted they were performed without pain. I know the operations were performed in the year 1842; my brother, Wm. H. Thurmond, had charge of the academy that year, and it was the only time I was a pupil in the academy. August 21st, 1849.

Andrew J. Thurmond

In addition to Mr. Venable's and Andrew J. Thurmond's, I present the certificates of E. S. Rawls and Wm. H. Thurmond, who were present, and witnessed one or both operations.

Georgia)
Clarke Co.)

I, Edmund S. Rawls, of Rome, Floyd county, Ga., on oath depose and say that I resided with my father in Jackson county, Ga., the year 1842, and was a pupil of Wm. H. Thurmond who then had charge of the Academy in the village of Jefferson. During that year I frequently inhaled sulphuric ether for its exhilarating effects in the office of Dr. C. W. Long and at other places in the village of Jefferson, and was well acquainted with the smell of ether and the effects of its inhalation.

On one occasion during that time I was present with James M. Venable in the office of Dr. C. W. Long in Jefferson, Jackson county, Ga., and witnessed Dr. C. W. Long cut out a tumour from the side of the neck of J. M. Venable while said Venable was full under the effects of the vapor of S. Ether inhaled from a towel and without his exhibiting the least symptoms of suffering pain from the operation. After the tumour was removed J. M. Venable was so unconscious from the operation having been performed that he would not believe the tumour was removed until it was shown him by Dr. C. W. Long.

Mr. Venable asserted that he was entirely unconscious of the performance of the operation and did not feel the least pain from its performance. This operation I am positive was performed during the year 1842 while I was a pupil of Wm. H. Thurmond as it was the only year he had charge of the academy in Jefferson. I am not positive I was present when Dr. C. W. Long removed the second tumour from the neck of J. M. Venable but if not present I recollect distinctly hearing him say soon after the tumour was removed that it was cut out while he was under the anaesthetic effect of S. Ether and that he did not suffer pain from the operation.

I conversed with J. M. Venable frequently during the year 1842 and he uniformly asserted that he did not suffer pain from the operations.

Sworn to and subscribed before me
this 2nd November, 1853
E. L. Newton, J. J. C.

            E. S. Rawls

         Atlanta, DeKalb Co., Ga.,
           April 3rd, 1853

C. W. Long, M.D.

It affords me pleasure to certify and I do hereby affirm

that I saw you perform an operation upon James M. Venable, to wit, the cutting out and removing of a tumor from the neck of the said James M. Venable.

The operation was performed when Mr Venable was under the *influence of sulphuric ether* produced by inhaling the same. I was intimate with Mr. Venable at the time of the operation; and afterwards frequently conversed with him upon the subject and he often told me that the operation produced no pain. The operation was performed in the town of Jefferson, Jackson County, Georgia, in the year *One Thousand Eight Hundred and Forty Two*.

Yours, Etc.,
Wm. H. Thurmond.

My third experiment in etherization was made on the third of July, 1842, and was on a negro boy, the property of Mrs. S. Hemphill, who resides nine miles from Jefferson. The boy had a disease of a toe, which rendered its amputation necessary, and the operation was performed without the boy evincing the least sign of pain. I present Mrs. Hemphill's statement of the report the boy gave her of the operation on his return home, which I conceive is sufficient on this point.

Georgia   )
Jackson Co.)

I, Sabrey Hemphill, certify that some six or seven years ago, I sent my negro boy, Jack, to Dr. C. W. Long to have his toe examined and cut off if necessary. The boy was sent some time during the summer and on the sabbath. After the boy returned home he informed me that Dr. Long cut off his toe and that he did not suffer any pain from the operation. The boy was sent in charge of his father.
Sept. 15th, 1849.

(Signed) Sabrey Hemphill.

Achievement

These were all the surgical operations performed by me during the year 1842, upon patients etherized; no other case occurring in which I believed the inhalation of ether applicable. Since '42 I have performed one or more surgical operations annually, on patients in a state of etherization.

The question will no doubt occur, why did I not publish the results of my experiments in etherization soon after they were made? I was anxious, before making my publication, to try etherization in a sufficient number of cases to fully satisfy my mind that anesthesia was produced by the ether, and was not the effect of the imagination, or owing to any peculiar insusceptibility to pain in the persons experimented on.

At the time I was experimenting with ether there were physicians "high in authority," and of justly distinguished character, who were the advocates of mesmerism, and recommended the induction of the *mesmeric state* as adequate to prevent pain in surgical operations. Notwithstanding thus sanctioned, I was an unbeliever in the science, and of the opinion, that if the mesmeric state could be produced at all, it was only on "those of strong imagination and weak minds," and was to be ascribed solely to the workings of the patient's imaginations. Entertaining this opinion, I was the more particular in my experiments in etherization.

Surgical operations are not of frequent occurrence in a country practice, and especially in the practice of a young physician; yet I was fortunate enough to meet with two (additional) cases in which I could satisfactorily test the anaesthetic power of ether. From one of these patients I removed three tumours the same day: the inhalation of ether was used only in the second operation, and was effectual in preventing pain, while the patient suffered severely from the extirpation of the other tumours. In the other case I amputated two fingers of a negro boy: the boy was etherized during one amputation, and not during the other; he suffered from one operation, and was insensible during the other. I have procured the certificates of the lady from whom the tumours were removed and her husband who was present and witnessed the operations; and also that of the owner of the boy, establishing the fact of the insensibility of the patients to pain during these operations. These certificates were procured in preference to those establishing other operations, because they not only show that the experiments were continued from year to year, but also show that they were conducted so as to test the power of etherization.

Georgia   )
Jackson Co.)

    I certify that sometime during the summer of 1843, Dr. C. W. Long cut out three wens from my head. He gave me some medicine to inhale, while cutting out one of the wens, and I suffered no pain from the operation. The pain was severe from the cutting out of the other wens.

Sept. 17, 1849
Test.
Thomas L. Stapler

                      (Signed) Mary Vinson

State of Georgia)
Jackson County)

    Personally appeared before me, Thomas L. Stapler, one of the acting Justice of the Peace of said county, Mary Vinson, who being duly sworn, deposeth and sayeth that the certificate is true which I gave to Dr. C. W. Long in the year 1849 in Regard to his cutting out three tumours from my head before cutting out one of them he gave me some medicine to inhale and I felt no pain at the time this operation was performed but suffered severely during the cutting out of the others which were taken out without being under the influence of the medicin.

Sworn to and subscribed before me
this 12th day December, 1853.
Thomas L. Stapler, J.P.

                        Mary Vinson

Georgia   )
Jackson County)
   I do hereby certify that I was present and saw William Vinson sign the certificate with his wife Mary Vinson, and that it was in his last illness in the year 1849, and that he died shortly thereafter.
December the 12th day, 1853
Thomas L. Stapler, J.P.

Georgia   )
Jackson County)
   I, Green L. Thompson, certify that I was present and witnessed Dr. C. W. Long, in the year 1845, cut off two fingers of a negro boy Isam, the property of my father in law, Ralph Baily, Sen. Before cutting off one of the fingers, Dr. C. W. Long gave the boy Isam, Sulphuric Ether to inhale from a towel or cloth, and while under the influence of the ether, cut off the finger without the boy showing the least sign of suffering pain. I have also heard the boy speak of the operation since and he always asserted that he did not feel the least pain when the operation was performed. The other finger was cut off without the boy being under the effects of the ether and the operation was painful. The operation was performed without any attempt to conceal the nature of the article used. Dr. C. W. Long stated that the article used was S. Ether. I had previously seen S. Ether inhaled, and from the smell and effects, know it was Sulphuric Ether inhaled by the boy Isam.
Sworn to and subscribed
before me this 2nd March 1854.
N. H. Pendergrass, N.P.
G. L. Thompson

   After fully satisfying myself of the power of ether to produce anaesthesia, I was desirous of administering it in a severer surgical operation than any I had performed. In my practice, prior to the published account of the use of ether as an anaesthetic, I had no opportunity of experimenting with it in a capital operation, my cases being confined, with one exception, to the extirpation of small tumors, and the amputation of fingers and toes.

I have stated that ether was frequently inhaled in this and some of the adjoining counties, for its exhilarating effects; and although I am conscious I do not deserve any credit for introducing its use for that purpose, yet as others, through their friends, have claimed to be the first to shew its safety, most of the certificates I have obtained establish the fact of its frequent inhalation for its exhilarating effects. I met with R. H. Goodman, who was present the night ether was first inhaled in Jefferson, and who removed to Athens, and introduced its inhalation in that place, and present his certificate. All the young gentlemen who were present the night I first administered ether, with one exception, are living, and their certificates can be procured, if necessary.

I certify that on the first of January, 1842, I resided in Jefferson, Jackson county, Georgia, and that about that time myself with other young men were in the habit of meeting at Doct. C. W. Long's Shop, and other rooms in the village and inhaling ether which he administered to us. We took it for its exhilarating effects. On the 20th of January of the same year, I removed to Athens in the above named state, where I introduced the inhalation of ether.

I and several of my young associates frequently assembled ourselves together and took it for the excitement it produced. After that I know it became very common to inhale ether in Athens, and that it was taken by a great many persons in the place, and was frequently taken in the college campus and on the street.
August 4th, 1849.
    R. H. Goodman,
    of the firm of Matthews, Goodman & Co.
    of Athens, Ga.

I have now in a very concise manner, presented a "plain, unvarnished" account of some of my experiments in etherization, and have said nothing of the comparative merits of ether, and the other anaesthetics, because that was foreign to my present subject. Had I been engaged in the practice of my profession in a city, where surgical operations are performed daily, the discovery, no doubt, would have been confided to others, who would have assisted in the experiments; but occupying a different position, I acted differently, whether justifiable or not.

While cautiously experimenting with ether, as cases occurred, with the view of fully testing its anaesthetic powers, and its applicability to severe as well as minor, surgical operations, others, more favorably situated, engaged in similar experiments; and consequently the publication of etherization did not "bide my time." This being the case, I leave it with an enlightened medical profession, to say, whether or not my claim to the discovery of etherization is forfeited, by not being presented earlier, and with the decision which may be made, I shall be content.

Dr. Long read an abridged edition of this paper before the meeting of the Medical Association of Georgia in 1852, concluding with: "I know that I deferred the publication too long to receive any honor from the priority of the discovery, but having by the persuasion of friends presented my claims before the profession, I prefer that its correctness be fully investigated before the medical society. Should the society say that the claim, though well founded, is forfeited by not being presented earlier, I will cheerfully respond, 'So mote it be'."

Following the reading of the paper, the Association adopted this resolution: "Resolved, That this society is of the opinion that Dr. Crawford W. Long was the first person who used Sulphuric Ether as an anesthetic in operations, and as an act of justice to him individually and to the honor of the profession of our own State, we most earnestly recommend him to present at once his claims to priority in the use of this most important agent to the consideration of the American Medical Association at its next meeting." Dr. Dickinson, Dr. Cooper, Dr. S. N. Harris, Committee.

Later, Dr. Long was informed that the American Medical Association could not take action in such matters, although at its meeting in 1870, the Association violated this policy, and adopted a resolution declaring Horace Wells to be the discoverer of anesthesia. At the meeting two years later, however, a motion to reaffirm this resolution, was laid on the table, as shown in the chapter entitled "Ether Controversy Retold."

Two notes by Dr. Paul F. Eve, Editor, were subjoined to Long's article published in the *Southern Medical Journal*, the first of which read as follows:

A few months ago, Dr. Long informed us of his early attempts at etherization, in Surgery. He was then informed that any claim set up at this late day to priority of discovery, would be severely criticized, if not violently resisted; and he had best, therefore, do all he could to fortify his position. He has accordingly sent us a number of certificates, properly attested; but as it is unusual for medical journals to admit these, and as besides, in our profession, the word of a gentleman is sufficient on all points of controversy, these are of course omitted here. We state, however, they may be seen by anyone curious in the matter, and their character may be judged by the *two following*, bearing most pointedly on the subject under discussion.

We have only to add, that the writer of this communication is a highly worthy member of the medical profession, exceedingly modest in his pretensions, and entitled to full credit for all he advances.

The "two following" certificates referred to are those of James Venable and Andrew J. Thurmond. The other certificates published in this reproduction of Long's article are the ones banned by Dr. Eve, a remarkable inconsistency. The second note added to the article says: "Our friend, Dr. Long, can lay no claim to the introduction of sulphuric ether as an exhilarating agent when its vapour is inhaled."

This statement is in direct contrast with the attitude taken by Dr. Eve at a later date, when he became a most enthusiastic supporter of Long and his claims, and urged him to present his cause before the American Medical Association. Dugas, the exponent of mesmerism, who succeeded Eve as editor of the *Southern Medical and Surgical Journal*, also at first opposed Long's claim vigorously, but subsequently became one of his advocates. One reason that these fellow Georgians did not support Long in the beginning was that, when they adopted inhalation anaesthesia, they chose chloroform instead of ether, a preference which long held sway in the warmer South. The position of Eve and Dugas in regard to Long is well brought out by Krafka.[24] It often "goes against the grain" for older men to recognize and admit the accomplishments of members of a younger generation, and they may be loath to encourage or assist them. J. C. Warren[25] stated that "the introduction of ether into surgical operations was done by my hands," while Seale Harris[26] has this to say about the discovery of insulin:

"Professor MacLeod, with his background of scientific training in the great laboratories of Leipzig and Berlin, was profoundly imbued with ideals of the German *geheimeraths*. He believed that heads of departments should receive the principal credit for researches which had been carried out in their laboratories, even if they themselves had not initiated, directed, or actively participated in the experiments. He was convinced that reports of his subordinates' achievements should be made by him, not by the subordinates. Acting on this belief, he made a number of reports, both spoken and written, which (perhaps unintentionally) gave his hearers and readers the impression that J. J. R. MacLeod was the principal discoverer of insulin, and that Frederick G. Banting and Charles H. Best were merely two among a number of assistants who had happened to work under his direction."

In this connection one is reminded of Thiersch's remark about Lister, whose contribution of antiseptic surgery came twenty-five years later (1867): "Lister's discovery, like all great discoveries, passed through the usual three stages: the first, when the world smiles and shakes its head, and says, 'That's all nonsense'; the second, when, with a shrug of the shoulders, and a look of contempt, it sneers, 'It's the merest *humbug*'; and finally, 'Oh, that's an old story, we knew that long ago.' (Dr. Warren anticipated this when he exclaimed of Morton's demonstration, 'This is no humbug.') Or, as James G. Mumford wrote of the fiery John Hunter, England's second famous name in surgery, 'No great man's contemporaries ever become his followers. Maturity does not seek novelty. The prophet must have young men around him if his words are not to fall fruitless.'"

5

COMMENT

THE FOREGOING PAPER BY DR. Long, with its documents and dates, is abundant proof that he administered the first anesthetic for a surgical operation, and used it in at least five operations before it was so used by any one else. Drugs by mouth and attempted anesthesia by mesmerism and the other methods of alleviating pain cannot be considered as successful since none of them stood the test of time. It is asserted here, with profound deference to the distinguished members of the medical profession who have expressed themselves otherwise, that Crawford Long's administration of ether to James Venable, March 30, 1842, accompanied by the removal of a tumor on his neck, without causing pain, constituted the discovery of surgical anesthesia. To attempt to explain that "discover" means more than it says is merely playing with the word. To discover is to find. Others had suggested that painless surgery could be done, but Long was the first person actually to do it. The greatest eloquence and richest poetry have been expended to describe the importance and value of anesthesia, but all language is futile in such an undertaking. Let us be content to characterize it as divine, a gift from on high.* The multitudes who have experienced its beneficent effects will endorse this description. Whether or not Long's achievement contributed anything to establishing universal anesthesia will be discussed later.

Since the event apparently passed off quite smoothly, doubtless the small group of young laymen present could not realize and appreciate the significance of what had happened, but not so with the principal actor, twenty-six-year-old Dr. Crawford Long. It has been charged that *he* did not appreciate it and became discouraged, and ignored anesthesia the rest of his life. Nothing could be further from the truth. Why should a physician with his academic and medical training not comprehend the importance of what he had done? Less than twelve months previously he had completed four years of study and observation among the leading surgeons of two of the largest cities, Philadelphia and New York. There he had seen surgery at its best for the times, and with his intelligence and sympathy he was bound to be impressed by the desperate need for means to obviate the agony attending operative procedures. Of course he was not aware of all the possibilities which anesthesia opened to surgery, and neither was any one else. Who then could have predicted the advanced surgery of today? But Dr. Long knew full well what his discovery meant for the surgery of the middle of the nineteenth century, which was that amputations, ligations, cystotomies, the removal of superficial tumors, and the reduction of fractures and dislocations could be done painlessly. That was true appreciation of the discovery of anesthesia for the times.

* Winston Churchill, English statesman, is quoted by the *Florida Times-Union*, September 11, 1947, as saying in a speech, "Medical science ought to create its saints. The world could do with 'the good Saint Anesthesia,' and the 'chaste and pure Saint Antiseptic.' "

But suppose James Venable's operation had not terminated so smoothly. There is no mention of pre-operative preparation; suppose the patient had vomited from a full stomach, and some of the food had lodged in the windpipe. Other unfavorable possibilities suggest themselves, but they did not happen, so we pass them. The consequences of an untoward or fatal result would have been too serious to contemplate. Manifestly, fate and the Lord decreed that Crawford Long should be successful that day.

The first anesthetic marked an epoch in history, both medical and civil. What was the reaction of the medical profession and populace in and around Jefferson when news spread of the unparalleled, almost unbelievable event? The favored witnesses of the operation must have been overcome with amazement, and probably gave vent to vociferous congratulations to the courageous young surgeon. As the surrounding country was sparsely inhabited and the number of practicing physicians correspondingly small, reports of the anesthetic spread slowly among the doctors. At the same time Dr. Long made no secret nor mystery of what he had done, and spoke of it freely to every one he met. It was natural for such an unprecedented procedure to receive unfavorable and violent criticism. Mrs. Taylor wrote of her father that he was considered reckless, perhaps mad. It was rumored throughout the country that he had a strange medicine by which he could put people to sleep and carve them to pieces without their knowledge. Some of his friends pleaded with him to abandon its use fearing that if an accident occurred when it was being administered, he might be mobbed and perhaps killed.

The physicians "high in authority" mentioned by Long were two nationally known men, **Paul F. Eve** and **L. D. Dugas**, both professors of surgery in the Medical College of Georgia, in Augusta, and both editors of the *Southern*

Medical and Surgical Journal. Eve preferred chloroform to ether as an anesthetic, while Dugas was one of America's principal exponents of mesmerism and had reported many operations performed under this method of anesthesia. These men were older than Crawford Long and far better known at the time, so that their delay in according recognition led him to hesitate in publishing his success with surgical anesthesia. It can be understood how a fledgling like Long would defer reporting such a radical innovation, especially with two of the leading practitioners of the state as censors. However, in 1848, two years after the demonstration at the Massachusetts General Hospital, Dr. Eve invited Dr. Long to Augusta, the object being to confer with him in order to prosecute his claims before the world as to his priority in the use of anesthesia.

Dr. R. J. Massey, who at the time was a student in the Medical College of Georgia (now the Medical School of the University of Georgia), gave the following account of Dr. Eve's introduction of Long, as published by Mrs. Taylor:

Young gentlemen, this is the event of a life-time. I introduce no distinguished individual. Our guest comes today unheralded. No great honors are heaped upon his head. He is a plain practical doctor. He comes, however, well equipped for the duties of his profession. He is learned, painstaking and very observant. His researches so far have already convinced the profession that a bright and useful life is before him. While quiet and diffident, he possesses all the requisites of success. He has already mastered a scientific solution that when properly learned will entirely revolutionize the field of surgery. I introduce to you Dr. Crawford W. Long, of Jefferson, whom posterity will honor as the very first man to apply practical anesthesia successfully to surgical operations. A Wells, a Morton or a Jackson, or Sir James Y. Simpson, the world renowned Scotch obstetrician, may for the present wrest the honors from Dr. Long. I will not live to see the time, but young gentlemen under the sound of my voice will see Dr. Long crowned as the greatest benefactor to suffering humanity. To him will be erected a monument of love and honor in grateful hearts, all over the world, while with heart-felt emotion I greet our guest and congratulate you upon the honor of this acquaintance with a brother doctor to whom the future is bright indeed.

THE WILHITE INCIDENT

No story about Crawford Long is complete without reference to what is known as the "Wilhite incident," and it is important because it led to the first nation-wide publication of Long's use of anesthesia. In 1876, Dr. P. A. Wilhite, of Anderson, South Carolina, consulted the celebrated Dr. Marion Sims,[27] in New York City, about his daughter, and was told that it would be necessary for her to be operated upon under ether. After the operation Dr. Wilhite told Dr. Sims that he had assisted in the first operation in which ether had been administered. "How could that be?" said Dr. Sims; "you have never been in Boston, and the first operation ever performed under ether was by Warren, of Boston, in October, 1846, or as some claim, by Marcy, of Hartford, in January, 1845." Dr. Wilhite then stated that he had assisted Dr. Crawford W. Long, of Georgia, in extirpating a tumor from the neck of Mr. Venable, in March, 1842, while he was completely anesthetized by the inhalation of sulphuric ether, and that Mr. Venable was as profoundly anesthetized as the patient then lying before them. He also said that he assisted Dr. Long to operate on other patients under the influence of ether in 1843 and 1844, while he was a student of medicine in Long's office. He declared that Long was the real and original discoverer of anesthesia, and he believed he would be so acknowledged if all the facts in the case were fully set forth.

Dr. Wilhite then spoke of the "ether frolics" in and around Jefferson and Athens, and said that in 1839 he had met several young people at Mr. Ware's, about five miles west of Athens, at a quilting. The girls and boys all finished the evening by inhaling ether. During the fun Wilhite spied a Negro boy at the door, who seemed to be enjoying the sport. He was invited to come in and take some ether, but refused. After he had refused several times the boys held him down while Wilhite poured some ether on a handkerchief and pressed it firmly over his mouth and nose. He fought furiously. They persisted and after a long struggle the boy became quiet and unresisting. The young men then let him alone. They were greatly surprised, however, when he did not get up immediately, and say or do some foolish thing for them to laugh at. His breathing was labored, and he could not be roused. Then they became greatly alarmed, and sent one of their number on horseback for Dr. Sydney Reese, at Athens, five miles distant. The messenger rode with all possible speed. He fortunately found Dr. Reese, who lost no time in going to Mr. Ware's. On his arrival he found the Negro lying on his back still soundly asleep. Young Wilhite, and his principal accomplice, thinking that they in mere play had murdered a fellow being, were so alarmed that they contemplated making their escape from the country; but the timely arrival of Dr. Reese soon restored their courage. Dr. Reese heard what had happened. He then threw water in the face of the sleeping Negro, slapped him, raised him up, shook him violently, and after a while brought him back to consciousness, to the great relief of all present. The doctor then gave the youngsters a lecture on the dangers of such frolics, and cautioned them against a repetition of their heedless act. This scare of course broke up the ether frolics in this neighborhood.

Dr. Wilhite told Dr. Sims that he thought Dr. Long got the idea of the possibilities of ether anesthesia from this occurrence, but Long was not present at the time, and did not move to Jefferson until 1841, two years after the incident. Later Dr. Long stated that he had never heard of the affair, and that Wilhite was mistaken about the time he entered his office, which was more than two years after Long had done his first operations under ether. As a matter of fact, Dr. Long said that although Wilhite studied in his office, he never assisted him in any operation, and later Wilhite admitted it, and explained that he had gotten his dates mixed, writing Long a letter to this effect. The account of the Negro boy, although strenuously disputed by Dr. Long's family, furnished the stimulus for Dr. Marion Sims' historical paper, the first to announce to the nation that Crawford Long was the discoverer of modern surgical anesthesia. The incident is cleared in the next two papers which were published substantiating Long's priority in surgical anesthesia, the articles by Grandy[28] and Young.[29]

Another story, also denied by Dr. Long's daughters, declared that his first operation on James Venable was not performed in his office, but under the mulberry tree by the side of the house. This does not sound reasonable, in the windy month of March, but many people still believe it. Everybody should be satisfied, however, by an old photograph recently found in Dr. Long's effects which shows the location of his office under the large mulberry tree.

6

MORE PROOFS

DR. LONG'S PAPER HAS BEEN criticized for not giving the dates of two operations which he performed before October, 1846, the operation on Mary Vinson for removal of three tumors from her head, and the one on Isam Bailey for amputation of two fingers. This oversight cannot be explained, but evidently Long gave the dates to Dr. Charles T. Jackson when he visited Athens, March 8th, 1854, because in Jackson's article on the "First Practical Use of Ether in Surgical Operations," in the *Boston Medical & Surgical Journal* April 11th, 1861, Jackson gives the date of the operation on Mary Vinson as September 9, 1843; and the operation on Isam Bailey as January 8, 1845.

There is no exact date for the sixth operation performed by Long before October, 1846, for which a certificate is presented:

Georgia   )
Floyd County)

I, Mary E. Ware, of Floyd County, Ga. certify that while residing near the village of Jefferson, in Jackson Co.,

Ga. Dr. C. W. Long extracted a tooth for me while under the influence of Sulphuric Ether, produced by the inhalation of the same from a towel or handkerchief, and without my suffering the least pain at the time the tooth was drawn. According to the best of my recollection and belief, the tooth was extracted in the summer of the year 1846. I am positive it was extracted by Dr. C. W. Long before I ever heard or saw any account of any other person using Sulphuric Ether for the purpose of preventing pain in the extraction of teeth or in the performance of any surgical operation.

February the 15, 1854.

Mary E. Ware

In her book on the life of her father, Mrs. Taylor states that he performed eight operations under ether before October, 1846, and Dr. Hugh Young of the Johns Hopkins Hospital, gives the same number. Long wrote that he did two operations annually for about four years, between 1842 and 1846, which would add up to eight, but certificates for only six have been found. Mrs. Eugenia Long Harper, last surviving child of Dr. Long, wrote the present author that she and all her sisters had often heard their mother say that her second baby, who was Mrs. Taylor herself, had been delivered by Dr. Long, under ether anesthesia. Mrs. Taylor also mentioned this fact, but according to Mrs. Harper, she would not give the date, nor the name of the baby, because, in so doing, the proud Mrs. Taylor would have divulged her own age. The date was December 27, 1845, which was more than a year prior to the ether anesthetic administered by James Y. Simpson* in England, who is credited with giving the first anesthetic in obstetrics. It is not presumed that Long included this delivery among his

---

* Simpson later used chloroform.

More Proofs 61

eight cases of surgical anesthesia. Records were kept inadequately in those days, and many were lost, a fact which was especially true of the important papers concerning Crawford Long's discovery of ether anesthesia. In fact, some of the documents travelled over the country several times, and once to Europe, for the inspection of those who were interested in them. In spite of the careful attention given these valuable possessions some easily could have been lost during the wide-spread confusion of the war and post-war years, as depicted so vividly in Margaret Mitchell's *Gone With The Wind*.

The exact number of persons who saw Long's first operation under anesthetic is not known, but the scene usually is shown with four witnesses. Of these the certificates of three have been presented: A. J. Thurmond, E. S. Rawls, and W. H. Thurmond. The fourth is signed by J. E. Hays, who saw the second operation on James M. Venable:

Georgia   )
Jackson County)

I, James E. Hays, of the County and State afore said, do state that I was a pupil in the Academy in the Village of Jefferson, Jackson county, Georgia, in the year 1842, then under the charge of William H. Thurmond. Sometime during that year, I was present in the office of Dr. C. W. Long, then of Jefferson, but now of Athens, Georgia, and witnessed the said Dr. Long cut a tumour or wen from the neck of James M. Venable, now deceased, while the said Venable was under the influence of Sulphuric Ether, produced by the inhalation of the same. The said James M. Venable seemed entirely unconscious of the performance of the operation, and insensible to pain until an instant before the operation was finished.

The operation required some time for its performance. I know I cannot be mistaken in the year the operation was performed, nor in the fact that it was Sulphuric Ether inhaled by said Venable. I had previously and frequently seen Sulphuric Ether inhaled and was well acquainted with its smell. I think there was but little difference in my age and that of said James M. Venable; we were both at that time about the age of twenty-one years.

The operation was publicly performed and Dr. Long made no attempt to conceal the character of the article inhaled, nor made any request that the result of the operation should be kept secret. The operation witnessed by me was the second one performed by Dr. Long on said James M. Venable.

Previous to the performance of this operation, the said Venable informed me that Dr. C. W. Long had cut out another tumour from his neck, in the early part of the same year, while he was under the influence of the inhalation of Sulphuric Ether, and that he was totally unconscious of and entirely insensible to pain during the performance of the operation. He informed me that after the effects of the inhalation of the Sulphuric Ether had passed off, he could not believe the operation was over until Dr. Long exhibited the tumour to him.

The fact of Dr. Long's using the inhalation of Sulphuric Ether to prevent pain in surgical operations, was public and notorious in and near the village of Jefferson, Jackson county, Georgia, in 1842.

Sworn to and subscribed
before me, this the 6th
April, 1864.   James E. Hays
N. H. Pendergrass, J.P.   Maj. G. M.

The date of the second operation on James Venable does not appear in this affidavit, but in his paper Dr. Long gives it as June 6th, 1842, and this is the date which appears on the statement for services rendered. The bill for two operations has been criticized for its small amount, but the young doctor explained that the amount was made trivial to induce other patients to submit to operations under ether. The bill is reproduced, not to show how small it was, but to demonstrate again that on these dates two such operations were performed under ether. Since James Venable's name appears so frequently in this narrative, in which he plays next to the leading role, it is not amiss to record that he belonged to one of the principal families of the state, the Venable family which owns famous Stone Mountain, sixteen miles from Atlanta.

James Venable
  To Dr. C. W. Long, Dr.

1842		cts.
January 28th	Sulphuric Ether	.25
March 30	Ether and exsecting tumour	2.00
May 13	Sulphuric Ether	.25
June 6	Exsecting tumour	2.00

Georgia)
Jackson County)

I, P. F. Hinton, clerk of the superior court of said county, do certify that the above account is a correct copy of an original made in his Book for medical services for the year 1842.

Given under my hand and seal of office this 27th of March, 1851.

P. F. Hinton, Clerk S.

E. S. Ellis[30] writes that this bill is the only real evidence that Long's operation ever had been performed.

Dr. Ange DeLaperriere lived near Jefferson at this time. He was an exiled French nobleman and a cousin of Count de Trobiand, later General de Trobiand, of the United States Army during the War Between the States, and during the reconstruction period was commander at New Orleans. Dr. DeLaperriere has descendents still living in Georgia. At first he refused to investigate Crawford Long's report on his anesthesia, but later became one of his warmest friends and advocates, and submitted the following affidavit:

Georgia)
Jackson County)

    I, Ange DeLaperriere, M.D., do certify that I resided in Jefferson, Jackson County, Georgia in the year 1842, and that sometime in that year I heard James M. Venable, then of said state and county, now deceased, speak of Dr. C. W. Long, then of Jefferson, in the county of Jackson, Georgia, now of Athens, cutting two tumours from his neck while under the influence of the inhalation of Sulphuric Ether, without pain, or being conscious of the performance of the operation.

    I do further certify that the fact of Dr. C. W. Long using Sulphuric Ether by inhalation to prevent pain in surgical operations was frequently spoken of and notorious in the county of Jackson, State of Georgia, in the year 1842. I do further certify that the said James M. Venable was born and raised near Jefferson and was regarded as a young man of truth and veracity.

Sworn to and subscribed
before me this 30th of March
1854.

N. H. Pendergrass, J.P.   A. DeLaperriere, M.D.

    Documents like the following demonstrate that Dr. Long certainly did not keep secret his discovery of anesthesia, but broadcasted it by word of mouth at every opportunity before 1846. Affidavits by a well-known Athens physician, and the wife of another one, support this statement:

More Proofs

Athens, Georgia,
Aug. 10th, 1878.

This certifies that in the month of May, 1843, I was present and assisted Dr. R. D. Moore of this place in amputating a leg. He said to his three students (I being one): If I had thought of it before we left home I would have tried Dr. Long's discovery, producing insensibility by inhalation of Aether.

Attest   James Camak, M.D.
Asa M. Jenkins
Ordinary of
Clarke County, Georgia.

I do certify that Dr. Crawford W. Long of Jefferson, Jackson County, Georgia, advised my husband, Dr. Joseph B. Carlton, a resident of Athens, Ga., to try sulphuric ether as an anesthetic in his practice.

In November or December, 1844 in Jefferson, Ga. while on a visit to the place, and in the office of Dr. Long, my husband extracted a tooth from a boy who was under the influence by inhalation of sulphuric ether, without pain, the boy not knowing when it was done.

I further state that the fact of Dr. Long using sulphuric ether to prevent pain was frequently spoken of in the county of Jackson at this time, and was quite notorious.

Sworn to and subscribed before
June 29th, 1907   Frank Betts
F. Y. Allgood, N.P., Clarke County, Ga.
                           Mrs. Emma H. Carlton.

Three other documents confirm Crawford Long's use of ether anesthesia in surgery at this time:

Georgia, Jackson County

Personally appeared before me John G. Lindsey, who being duly sworn deposeth and sayeth that he was a classmate of James M. Venable in the Academy at Jefferson in Jackson County, Georgia, in the year 1842, then in charge of William H. Thurmond, Esq., and at some time during that year there was a surgical operation performed on James M. Venable by Dr. C. W. Long while as he (the said J. M. Venable) has repeatedly told me he was under the influence of sulphuric ether administered to him by the said Dr. Long. I recollect to have heard him (Venable) say often in conversation with others that the operation was performed without pain whatever. The operation was cutting a tumour or wen from the back of the said Venable's neck. As to the year above given I know I cannot be mistaken as it was the only year Mr. Thurmond ever had charge of the Academy at Jefferson.

Sworn to and subscribed before me the 12th day of December, 1853.

James H. Hayes, J.P.   John G. Lindsey.

A letter to "Miss Fannie Long," intended for Mrs. Francis Long Taylor, from E. S. Rawls, one of the witnesses of the first operation on Venable:

Marion, Perry Co., Ala.,
June 3, 1880.

Miss Fannie Long:

Your letter dated May 1, 1880, has just come to hand. I assure you that I have never received a letter from your father or anyone else relative to the subject you mention except about 1850. I received a letter and some interrogations which I filled to the best of my memory. In my native village, Jefferson, Jackson County, Georgia, it was a very common thing (in the year 1842 I was about sixteen years old) for a parcel of us town youngsters to meet together and take or inhale ether for sport. We bought what the druggist labeled sulphuric ether. Sometimes your father, Dr. C. W. Long would be with us. Occasionally some of us would get very much bruised but experienced no pain until after we recovered from the influence of the ether. Dr. Long frequently made expressions relative to the effects of ether on the system, he said that surgical operations could be performed without pain if enough ether would be used.

The doctor at that time was medicating a tumor on the neck of James M. Venable. He told Mr. Venable that he could cut out the tumor and that he (Venable) would suffer no pain. A few days after this conversation I accompanied Mr. Venable to Dr. Long's office. Dr. Long gave Venable some ether on a folded towel and Dr. Long cut out the tumor. Mr. Venable said he experienced no pain in the least. Mr. Venable and I were intimate friends and school mates at the time the above took place. You ask me what suggested the idea to his mind? He saw us get hurt while under the influence of ether. In other words he saw the apple fall, like Sir Isaac Newton he gave it his attention. You ask was his determination sudden. So far as I know it was, for soon after we began to use ether for sport he proposed to operate on Mr. Venable.

Your third question is: "Did he receive encouragement from any one?" Not that I know of.

Your fourth question: "Was it the deliberate conviction of his own mind?" In expression of ideas he made no quotations.

"Had we ever heard of any one being made insensible by the inhalation of ether before this time?" I had used it and saw a great many others use it as I have stated, but never saw it used for any other purpose than sport and amusement until I saw Mr. Venable take or inhale it. At that time Mr. Venable and I were going to a literary school. I did not go into any office to read medicine until the year 1853.

I will take pleasure in answering any questions or give any information in my power. I expect I am the only living witness to the operation performed on Mr. Venable by your father.

Most Respectfully,
E. S. Rawls.

You are at liberty to use this in any way you may see proper.

And finally a letter from Dr. John F. Groves, who was a student in Dr. Long's office in 1844-1845:

Cuhutta, Ga., Dec. 13, 1894.

Mrs. Frances Long Taylor,
Dear Madam:

In 1844, soon after I attained my majority, I decided to adopt medicine as my profession and began to think where and under whom I should begin the preparatory study. My father asked me to choose from among the number of physicians I knew the one I preferred to act as preceptor to me. Knowing Dr. Long so well and believing him to be a man of no ordinary ability, I at once fixed upon him as my choice. I entered Dr. Long's office in May, 1844, as the first student ever under his care. As I progressed with my studies he saw fit to make known to me his discovery by the use of which he could perform surgical operations without giving any pain to his patient. [Here follows a description of the first cases, but as he was not a witness to these, I do not quote him.]

Not satisfied, however, that there was not more to learn about this great discovery, he proposed that we test it further, personally, which we did in his office, where with closed doors we administered it to each other to prove its perfect anesthetic effect, also to discover any bad effect to the subject etherized. Owing to the prejudice and ignorance of the populace, Dr. Long was prevented from using ether in as many cases as he might have. Thus in the two years preceding my entering Dr. Long's office he had only

More Proofs

about six cases in which to try the anesthetic effects of ether.

The first case that came under his care where its use was applicable after my going into his office was not until January 8, 1845, which was the case of a negro boy having two fingers to amputate, caused by neglected burn. I, as the only student still with the doctor, he had me to accompany him to see the operation and assist in the administration of ether. The first finger was removed without pain, the second without ether, the child suffered extremely. This was done to prove that insensibility to pain was due to the agent used.

Soon after this in January, Dr. J. D. Long (a cousin) came into the office as a fellow student; later toward spring came P. A. Wilhite and in August came Dr. Long's brother, H. R. J. Long. We four remained there at Dr. Long's office as students until the opening of the fall term of the medical colleges.

(Signed) J. R. Groves, M.D.

Sworn and subscribed to and before me, Dec. 15, 1894.
Wm. H. Wilson, N.P.

Mrs. Taylor adds:

In a letter written to Dr. Hugh H. Young, of Baltimore, January 15, 1897, describing the operation performed upon the Negro boy, Dr. Groves says the patient was placed in a recumbent position, on a bed, with the hand to be operated on to the front for the convenience of the surgeon, and further continues:

Dr. Long poured ether on a towel and held it to the patient's nose and mouth too, to get the benefit of inhalation from both sources. Dr. Long determined when the patient was sufficiently etherized to begin the operation by pinching or pricking him with a pin. Believing that no harm would come of its use for a reasonable length of time he profoundly anesthetized the patient, then gave me the towel and I kept up the influence by holding it still to the patient's nose. The patient was entirely unconscious—no struggling—patient passive in the hands of the operator. After a lapse of fifty years you would hardly suppose that a man could remember every minute detail, but I have clearly in my mind all the facts I have given you.

Your obedient servant,
J. F. Groves, M.D.

The papers of Dr. Joseph Jacobs[31] include six other affidavits attesting to the operation on James Venable, under anesthesia, signed by Sarah Venable, his mother; John and Delilah Venable, Mary Jane Davis and Elizabeth Duke, his brother and sisters; Martha E. Pendergrass, Robert J. Millican, Joshua N. Glenn, and Joseph W. Allen, Camilla S. Few, James E. Hayes and Wyatt Wood.

Confirming the reliability of those whose names are signed to the documents presented, and of many whose statements are not herein reproduced, the following certificate is given, signed by the clerk and ordinary of Jackson county, the home of Crawford Long at the time of the first anesthestic. These people were among the best citizens of the community.

Georgia   )
Jackson County)

We, the undersigned P. F. Hinton, clerk of the Superior Court, and John G. Pittman, ordinary of said county, do certify that we are acquainted with the following named persons, and that we believe them to be entitled to credit, viz., James M. Venable, John Venable, Eliza Venable, Mrs. Sarah Venable, Elizabeth Liddell, Sam Davis, W. H. Thurmond, A. J. Thurmond, J. E. Hays, E. S. Rawls, C. L. Few, O. M. Lowery, G. M. D. Few, Joseph H. Davis, W. S. Thompson, I. N. Randolph, R. I. Millican, Esq., W. T. Millican, Esq., I. B. Nabors, Mrs. E. Nabors, N. H. Pendergrass, Esq., W. N. Barrett, Wm. Henderson, I. N. Glenn, Dr. A.

More Proofs

DeLaperriere, Dr. I. C. DeLaperriere, Ralph Bailey, Sr., Milton Bailey, G. L. Thompson, Dr. J. D. Long, Dr. P. A. Wilhite, Joseph H. Adams, Mrs. M. Ware, W. Vincent, Mrs. Mary Vincent, John Calahan, W. M. Duke, Wyat Wood, Jos. H. Hayes, J. G. Lindsey, A. I. Lindsey, J. C. Stanley, W. A. Worsham, and C. Witt, Esq. In witness whereof we have hereto set our hands and seal of office this 27th March, 1854.

P. F. Morton
John G. Pittman, Ordinary.

Certain authors refer to Long's operations as "minor." As surgical operations go today most of Long's operations might be classed as "minor," as may many of the operations which were performed in the eighteen-forties all over the world. However, experienced surgeons, like Hubert Royster,[32] declare that no surgical operation is minor. The gravity of an operation is not to be judged by the size of the part involved, nor by the amount of blood shed. Certainly the amputation of a finger should not be classed as a minor operation. If it is not done according to certain rules the patient may suffer a completely crippled hand the rest of his life, and who can overestimate the value of the human hand?

Authors speak in disparaging tones of the insignificant number of operations performed by Crawford Long, probably two a year between 1842 and 1846. This is not remarkably out of proportion for one young "country" general practitioner compared with the total number of operations performed by several nationally-known surgeons at the Massachusetts General Hospital, during approximately the same period. Quoting from Graham,[33] "Of course in 1846 there was no surgery in the modern sense. In fact there were no surgeons as we understand them today. No specialization in medical practice had occurred, and every doctor was a general practitioner. Even as late as 1880 when the American Surgical Association was founded by Gross, the original members were all general practitioners."

Russian and German surgeons, in World War I, reported many instances of the bradycardiac reaction of arteriovenous aneurysm, so that there was a tendency to call the syndrome "Wigdorowitsch's Sign," but Rudolph Matas,[34] pre-eminent in American surgery, insisted that the manifestation be known as "Branham's Sign," after Dr. Henry H. Branham, of Brunswick, Georgia, who first described it twenty-five years previously, in 1890, notwithstanding the fact that he never reported but one case. The work of the European surgeons in this regard may have constituted an independent discovery, but it is not impossible that they may have read or heard of Branham's one published article.[35] It seems reasonable to believe that the closer in time similar discoveries are revealed, the more likely they are to be independent. Proskauer[36] reported the independent discovery, in 1847, of rectal anesthesia by Dupuy and Pirogoff. The manuscript of the former was read before the National Academy of Medicine, in Paris, March 16, 1847, while Pirogoff's manuscript-letter was submitted before the same body, six weeks later, April 27, 1847. These are classed as independent discoveries. The four and one-half years intervening between Long's discovery of surgical anesthesia and Morton's demonstration in the same country allowed too much time to elapse for one to be sure that Morton's was an independent discovery. This is an idea to be elaborated under "Ether Controversy Retold."

It has been written that Long became discouraged in promoting his claims as the discoverer of ether anesthesia and abandoned the use of ether, but this statement fails to tally with the facts. In a letter to Dr. Garnett W. Quillian, dated August 30, 1921, Mrs. Taylor gave a list of her father's operations under ether anesthesia, between 1846 and 1878, that she could remember, or that were told her by persons who had knowledge of the procedures. She was sure that he had performed many more operations than these, but the books containing the records were lost after her brother's death in 1908. At the time she wrote to Dr. Quillian there were still living many witnesses of these operations. "Minor operations" made little impression on her, and she mentions only the cases in which the patient was in a dangerous condition. During the war years, between 1861 and 1865, when Long was appointed by the Governor of Georgia to treat surgical cases, he performed many operations under anesthesia, of which there is no record. He ministered to both Confederates and Federals. Also, for the year 1850, when he lived with his family in Atlanta, there is no account of the number of operations. Following is Mrs. Taylor's letter, in part:

1. 1847. Amputation of finger.
2. 1856. Amputation of a leg of a tenant.
3. 1857. Amputation of breast of Mrs. Williamson McCleskey. Professor Orr, formerly president of Martin Institute, in Jefferson, wrote as follows of this case:

About the year 1857 or 1858, there lived in Jackson county, near Jefferson, Mr. Williamson McCleskey. His wife, Mrs. Lucretia Weir McCleskey, had cancer of the breast. Dr. Crawford W. Long came from Athens, Georgia, to Jefferson, and brought with him to Mr. McCleskey's home, his cousin, Dr. David Long, to assist him. My mother, being a warm personal friend of Mrs. McCleskey, was asked to be present. Dr. David Long administered the sulphuric ether, and Dr. Crawford Long performed the operation successfully. I know these to be facts because my mother was present and gave me this information. Mrs. Lucretia Weir McCleskey lived to a vigorous old age, dying in her ninety-second year. At the time the operation was performed, Mrs. McCleskey was in her forty-third year.

(Signed) S. P. Orr

I also learned the above facts from my mother.

(Signed) Margery E. Orr.

Dr. David Long was one of Dr. Crawford Long's first medical students. He read medicine in Dr. Long's office in 1845 and 1846, and was trained by his preceptor to administer ether in surgery. Mr. and Mrs. Orr are almost positive that Mrs. McCleskey's operation was in 1857.

1862. Serious operation upon Mrs. S. P. Thurmond.

1867 or 1868. Dr. Long removed the breast (cancerous) of a lady from Jefferson, Georgia. She had been operated upon at a Surgical Institute. The cancer returned owing (Dr. Long said) to the fact that the glands under the arm had not been removed or the ribs scraped. This precaution he always used. I do not know what year his first removal of a cancerous breast occurred.

1869. This operation was successful, but it is not said which operation is meant. The patient died about 1875 from another disease. Soon afterward he amputated the breast for cancer of a lady from Madison, Georgia. When I asked my father his charge for this operation, his reply was one hundred dollars, but in New York the fee would possibly have been five hundred to one thousand dollars.

1870. Mrs. Howard Van Epps (well known to Georgians), serious operation.

1872. Mrs. Eliza Mandeville, several operations.

1872. Mrs. John McCalla, delivery.

1872. Mrs. Fannie Hudgins, delivery. (Dr. Long was the consulting physician, delivering her of twins. She was thoroughly anesthetized.)

1873. Mrs. Giles Mitchell, Removal of cancer.

1874. Oct. 10th. Mrs. Elizabeth Bussey. A very dangerous obstetrical case, very large child, delivered with instruments.

She told me that she was so thoroughly anesthetized that she was unconscious for an hour or more.

1875. Mrs. LeSeur. Removal of cancerous tumor from the groin. Her niece, Mrs. Matthews, with whom I have just conversed, described the patient's joy after arousing from unconsciousness that she felt no pain throughout the operation. She died in Atlanta forty years later.

1876. Mrs. Julia Dorough Long, delivery.

1876. Mrs. George Bancroft, delivery.

1877. Mrs. James Comer, delivery.

1877. Amputation of man's leg in Jackson county, Georgia.

1856. Amputation of leg of a tanner who had been poisoned in a vat.

My mother bore twelve children. Her first was born in 1843. I have heard her say that it was a terrible ordeal, but with later children my father administered ether to her so that child-bearing lost much of its terrors. All my life I have known and seen the effects of ether. I cannot remember when it was not familiar to me. When a girl, my father gave it to me in two slight operations.

(Signed) Frances Long Taylor.

Since this book was begun, Mrs. C. S. Bostwick, of Atlanta, phoned the author that when her mother, Mrs. James Russell, was born in Athens, in 1865, Dr. Crawford Long was called to give the anesthetic in the case, which was a very difficult one.

Thus we have record of at least twenty-one occasions after 1846 (seven obstetrical) when Long used ether in surgical operations. There must have been dozens of other cases during the thirty-two years from 1846 to the time of his death in 1878.

Probably a natural reason for hesitating to believe that Long could have given the first surgical anesthetic was the size and location of his home, Jefferson,* Georgia, but any reflection should immediately dispel the idea that such a thing could not happen there, no matter how far removed and isolated was the little village. Many of medicine's most important discoveries, and the world's greatest events, have occurred in such places, like the isolated army post in Michigan, where Beaumont began his historical work on the physiology of the stomach; or the canebrakes of Alabama, where Sims learned to save women from invalidism. And then it must be remembered that in the Gospel of St. John 1:46, Nathaniel asked could any good thing come out of Nazareth.

---

* Now a prosperous county-seat of 2,000 inhabitants.

7

ETHER CONTROVERSY RETOLD

IN 1920 THE ELECTORS OF THE New York University Hall of Fame* voted a place for William T. G. Morton as the discoverer of anesthesia. Some time later, that fine scholar and gentleman,** Dr. William H. Welch[37] wrote me a letter in long hand, in which he said that he believed his Ether Day Address of 1908, supporting Morton, was a strong factor in Morton's election. Dr. Welch, who himself was one of the electors, stated that he had sent a copy of his address to each of the others. Naturally they were impressed by arguments from such a distinguished source. What information they possessed concerning other claimants is not known.

In his paper Dr. Welch spoke of Crawford Long as follows: "While the accepted rule that scientific discovery dates from public demonstration is a wise one, we need not in this instance withhold from Dr. Long the credit of

---
* Not to be confused with National Statuary Hall in the Capitol at Washington.
** Professor W. D. Hooper of the University of Georgia said there used to be an unwritten rule in a South Carolina college that every member of the faculty must be *either* a scholar or a gentleman. Dr. Welch was both.

independent and prior experiment and discovery, but we cannot assign to him any influence upon the historical development of our knowledge of surgical anesthesia or any share in the introduction to the world at large of the blessings of this matchless discovery."

Sir William Osler[38] allowed Long no part at all in the introduction of surgical anesthesia, when he affirmed: "In science the credit goes to the man who convinces the world, not to the man to whom the idea first occurs. Morton convinced the world; the credit is his." Thus Umpires Welch and Osler have ruled Long out of the game; it is our purpose to reinstate him.

While advocates of Crawford Long as the discoverer were disappointed by the action of the electors, it provided the needed stimulus for trying to establish his rights to the coveted honor. In 1921, at a sectional meeting of the American College of Surgeons, in Atlanta, at the suggestion of Dr. E. C. Davis, chairman of the program committee, a paper on Long and his work was read and published,[39] culminating in the formation of the Crawford W. Long Memorial Association. In 1926, through the activities of this organization in sponsoring public subscriptions, Long's statue was erected in Statuary Hall, in the National Capitol, where it had been voted a place by the Georgia Legislature in 1902, which failed to provide funds for it. The instigator of this successful movement was Dr. Joseph Jacobs, prominent Atlanta pharmacist, who at sixteen years of age, had worked in Long's drug store in Athens. In his effort to promote the cause of his former employer, he was ably assisted by the late Richard B. Russell, Chief Justice of the Supreme Court of Georgia. Dr. Jacobs' admiration for Crawford Long knew no bounds, and he determined that he should receive the recognition he deserved.

All during my acquaintance with Dr. Jacobs he continued to observe: "They learned about anesthesia from Crawford Long," and he gave reasons for this belief to be explained later. We were so happy to have the statue at last put up in Washington that we must have felt that our mission was completed, and Jacobs' declaration seemed superfluous. It became rooted in my mind, however, as other ideas about the discovery of anesthesia have been forcibly brought to my attention, unsought. Then, in December, 1944, Dr. George H. Bunch,[40] of Columbia, South Carolina, recited to me the full revealing story of Dr. Charles T. Jackson, which I had not known before. I am yet to recover from the shock.

It is not the object of the present discussion to reflect unnecessarily upon any of the participants in the dramatic history of the discovery of anesthesia. In fact, it is hoped that a story may be unfolded which will assign an important and indispensable role to each actor in the chain of events. As Oliver Wendell Holmes wrote, "Everybody wants to have a hand in the great discovery." Since the priority of Long's use of surgical anesthesia is now generally accepted, the present objective is to disprove the assertions of Welch, Osler, and others that Long's accomplishment had no influence upon the historical development of our knowledge of anesthesia, and did not entitle him to "Share in the introduction to the world at large of the blessings of this matchless discovery."

Wells

No controversy in the annals of science concerning an important discovery has been given as much consideration as the discovery of surgical anesthesia. The original dispute as to who was the discoverer lay principally between William Thomas Green Morton, a dentist of Boston, and Charles Thomas Jackson, a physician and chemist of the same city. Horace Wells, Hartford dentist, usually is regarded as the first to use nitrous oxide gas in the extraction of teeth, in 1844, and for that reason he has been acclaimed by some as the discoverer of anesthesia. On account of his lamented death in 1848, his right was not pushed as vigorously in the Ether Controversy as that of the others. His employment of the gas in anesthesia had been successful until he attempted to demonstrate it in January, 1845, at the Massachusetts General Hospital, when the patient made a sharp outcry just as the tooth was drawn, and the audience hissed and drove Wells from the amphitheater. The patient admitted later that he had felt no pain, and thereafter the young dentist succeeded satisfactorily in the extraction of teeth under nitrous oxide gas, which, however, could not be considered adequate for surgical operations.

In 1864 the American Dental Association passed a resolution declaring Wells to be the discoverer of anesthesia. In this connection, the succeeding extract from a recent letter from Dr. Morris Fishbein, Editor of the *Journal of the American Medical Association*, is of interest:

In the Transactions of the American Medical Association, volume 21, 1870, page 63, appears the following statement: "On motion of Dr. H. R. Storer, of Massachusetts, it was Resolved, That the honor of the discovery of practical anesthesia is due to the late Dr. Horace Wells, of Connecticut."

The Transactions of 1872, volume 23, page 71, read: "The following, offered by Dr. Henry Hartshorne, of Pennsylvania, was *laid on the table*: Resolved, That reaffirming the resolution of 1870, by this Association, recognizing Horace Wells as the discoverer of the practical application of anesthesia for surgical purposes, we hereby acknowledge the goodwill and sense of justice evinced by Sir James Y. Simpson, and others in England, toward an American discoverer which led to originating in England of the

'Horace Wells Testimonial Fund,' and we cordially recommend a movement in this country for the same purpose."

MORTON

Dr. Morton was born in Charlton, Massachusetts, in 1819, being therefore four years younger than Crawford Long. Authors continue to reassert that Morton graduated in dentistry from the Baltimore College of Dental Surgery, the world's first dental school, founded in 1840, but a recent letter to the writer from J. Ben Robinson, dean of that institution, now the University of Maryland School of Dentistry, declares that Morton not only never graduated there, but never matriculated. In 1849, however, this institution granted him an honorary degree in dentistry, while in the same year the Baltimore College of Physicians and Surgeons conferred on him the degree of M.D. The medical course at Harvard at that time was two years. Morton attended lectures at Harvard from 1844 to 1846, but received no degree in medicine. Both he and Wells were capable dentists. Morton was five years younger, and studied dentistry under Wells. September 30, 1846, Morton administered ether to Eben Frost and successfully removed a tooth. Thus encouraged, he asked to be allowed by the authorities of the Massachusetts General Hospital to demonstrate a drug in the Bulfinch amphitheater which would prevent pain in surgical operations. He called the drug "letheon," which later was found out to be ether with aromatic substances added to disguise its odor.

Permission was granted Morton to try the anesthetic for the removal of a tumor on the neck of a young printer, Gilbert Abbott, and October 16, 1846, was set as the day for the operation. Morton was late in keeping his appointment and explained that he was detained awaiting the completion of a new inhaler. This is the excuse usually given for the delay, but Dr. Robert B. Osgood, prominent Boston surgeon, vouches for the following story which was related to me by my classmate, Dr. W. L. Moss, of Athens, Georgia, noted for his work in blood grouping:

Dr. Henry Jacob Bigelow, rising young surgeon, had made arrangements for the event, and had invited several leading Boston surgeons to be present. When Morton did not appear on schedule, Dr. John C. Warren, who was to perform the operation, became impatient, and was about to proceed without the assistance of Dr. Morton. Bigelow, fearing something was amiss, jumped into his cabriolet, and hurried to the dentist's office. There he found Morton packing a satchel preparatory to leaving town. Dr. Bigelow quickly persuaded him not to leave, and rushed the frightened young man to the amphitheater, where the celebrated procedure took place, without mishap. Morton was always noted for having plenty of self-confidence and should not be accused of having less because of this incident. A tremendous act was about to go on, in which he was to play the principal role, with a well-qualified and critical audience. And besides, he must have been thinking of Wells' unfortunate experience, which he had witnessed, in the same place, almost two years before. The occurrence of October 16 shows how much more aid was accorded Morton than Long, when each gave his first surgical anesthetic. In Morton's demonstration three surgeons, especially, deserve distinction along with Morton: Warren, for performing the operation; Bigelow, for arranging it, and publishing the result to the world; and later, George Hayward, for compelling Morton to expose the fact that "letheon" was only masked ether.

When Morton realized the magnitude of the demonstration and what it might mean to him in dollars and cents, he had the discovery patented, in the names of Morton and Jackson, which was an obvious admission of his indebtedness to Jackson for suggesting to him the idea of ether anesthesia.

The first sentence of the patent reads: "Be it known that *we*, Charles T. Jackson and William T. G. Morton, of Boston, county of Suffolk and State of Massachusetts, have invented or discovered a new and useful improvement in surgical operations."

The part claimed to have been played by Jackson will be discussed later. The pair planned to keep the identity of the agent a secret and sell rights to use it. Dr. Hayward forced Morton to expose the true nature of "letheon" by refusing to permit its use so long as its mystery continued. The patent turned out to be invalid, although in one instance Morton brought suit unsuccessfully against Dr. Charles A. Davis, superintendent of the United States Marine Hospital, at Chelsea, Massachusetts, for infringement. Jackson withdrew his name from the patent on condition that he be paid $500.00 and should receive ten per cent of the profits, another striking evidence of Morton's obligation to Jackson. If Morton's patent could have been maintained, his estimated share of the profits from rights to use it in the United States alone would have amounted to $355,000 in fourteen years, when the patent expired.[41]

Then, within a few days after Morton's demonstration, arose the famous "Ether Controversy," in which Morton, Jackson, and Wells each claimed to be the discoverer of anesthesia. Morton and Jackson agreed to become "co-discoverers," and the controversy began in earnest when Morton found out that Jackson had written the French Academy of Sciences, where he was well known, announcing himself alone to be the discoverer. Without mentioning Morton's name, Jackson added that he had employed a Boston dentist to give the anesthetic during a tooth extraction, and after this succeeded he had arranged for the dentist to administer ether again for a surgical operation, which also terminated with success.

When Morton learned these facts he sent a Memoir to the French Academy declaring that he was the discoverer of surgical anesthesia and that neither Jackson nor anyone else had much to do with it. A war of words and pamphlets ensued, with each contestant calling the others by uncomplimentary names. With all this Crawford Long had nothing to do, although he heard of it. After the conflict reached the Congress, in 1847, and the three claimants were exhausting their supply of accusations and epithets, United States Senator W. C. Dawson,* of Georgia, on April 15, 1854, arose and introduced the name of Crawford Long as the discoverer, and it was added to the others. This move is reported to have exploded a bombshell into the debate, but the dispute was by no means stopped. It raged intermittently on Congressional floors without a permanent decision from 1847 to 1863, so that it may be said that a Civil War** was required to end it. The object of the dispute was two-fold: to determine who was the discoverer of anesthesia; and mainly to decide who would receive the prize of $100,000, which later was raised to $200,000. The result was that no prize was awarded. Since the remainder of Morton's tumultuous life has but little bearing on the story of Crawford Long, the details will be omitted. The disappointed

* William Crosby Dawson (1798-1856), of Greensboro, Georgia, U. S. Senator from 1849 to 1855. Dawson county, Georgia, is named for him. Considerable research failed to reveal just *why Senator Dawson asked Jackson to visit Long*. It was said that Jackson was related to Dawson by marriage, but such a story could not be confirmed.

** In speaking of the American war of 1861-1865 objection is made to the time-honored designation of "Civil War" on the ground that a civil war is a conflict between parties in the same country. The United States was divided into two countries, with separate governments, so "War Between The States" is correct. For the sake of brevity it might be called the WBTS.

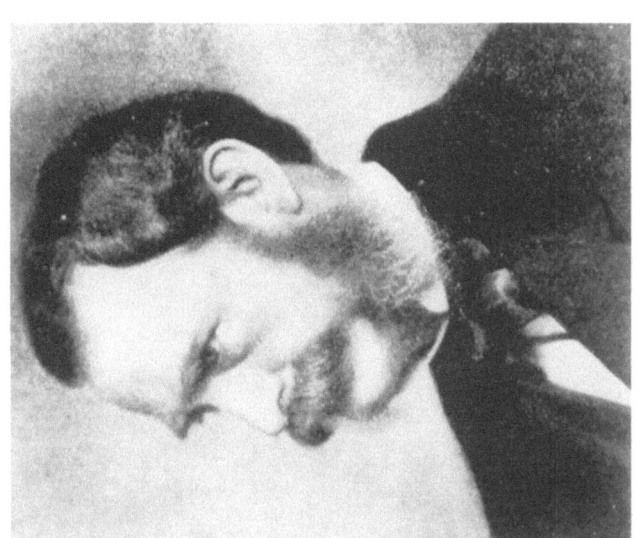

William H. Morton (1819-1868)
Courtesy Massachusetts General Hospital

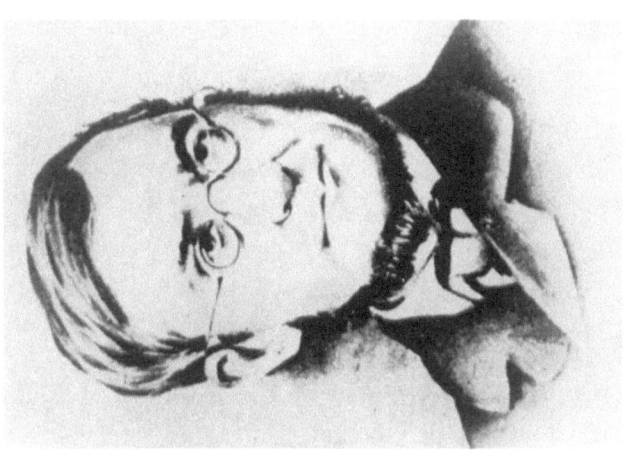

Charles T. Jackson (1805-1880)
From Hugh H. Young Collection

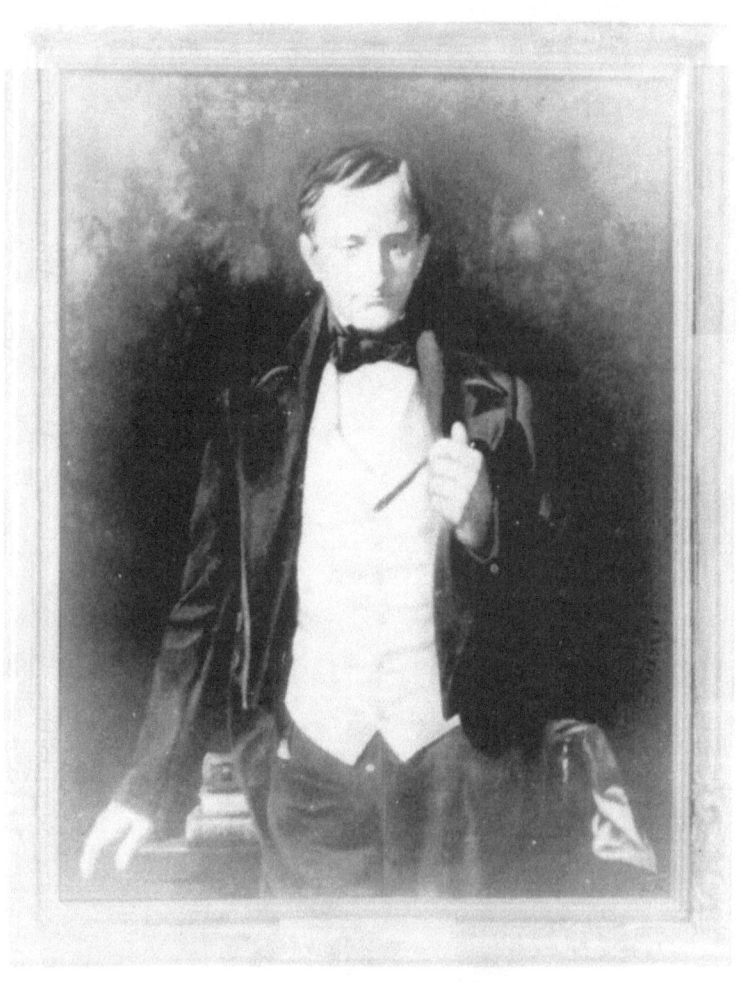

Crawford W. Long painted by Lewis Gregg, in Alumni Hall. The University of Georgia

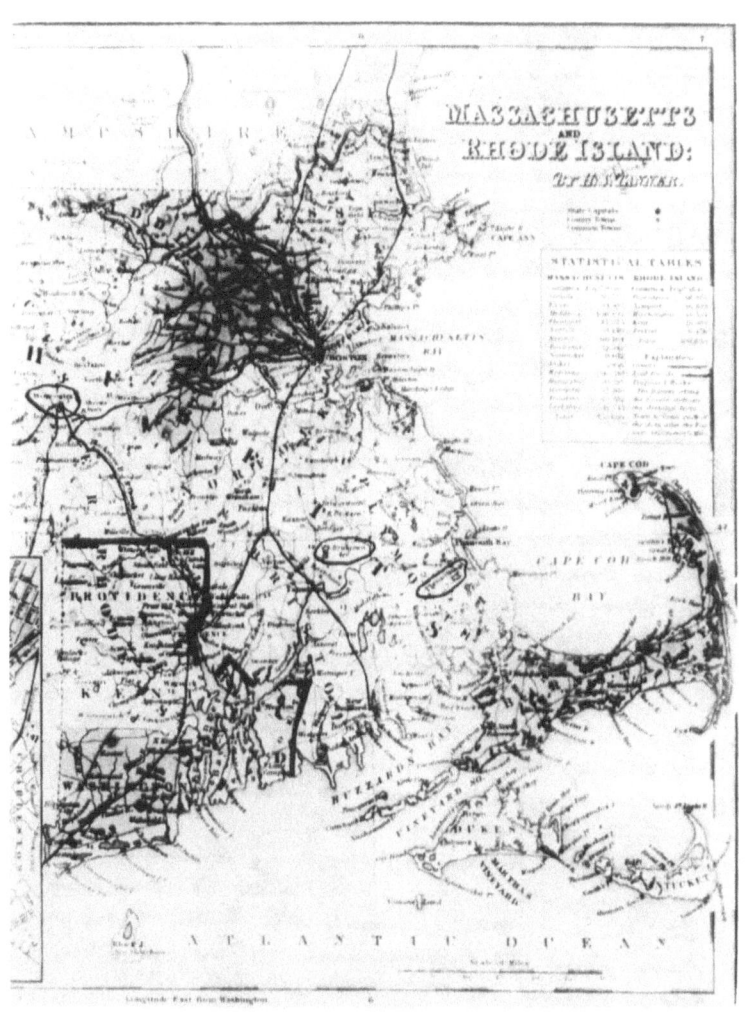

Eastern Massachusetts in 1841, showing relative locations of Plymouth, Bridgewater, and Boston

FACSIMILE OF MANUSCRIPT PAGE OF CRAWFORD WILLIAMSON
LONG FROM HIS ADDRESS READ BEFORE THE GEORGIA STATE
MEDICAL SOCIETY

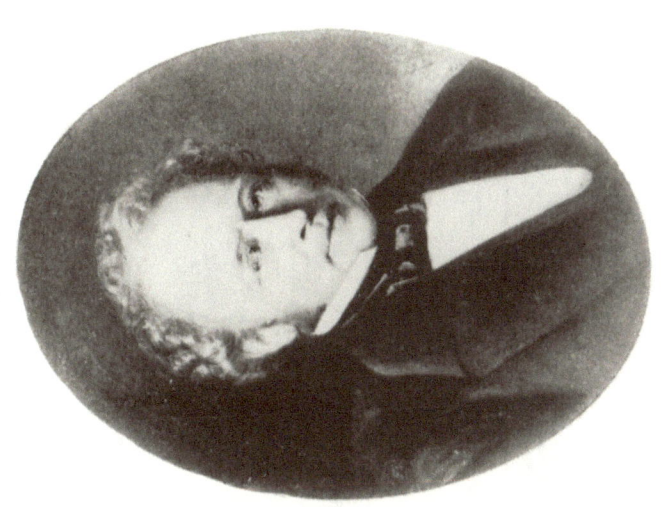

George Hayward (1791-1863)
Courtesy Massachusetts General Hospital

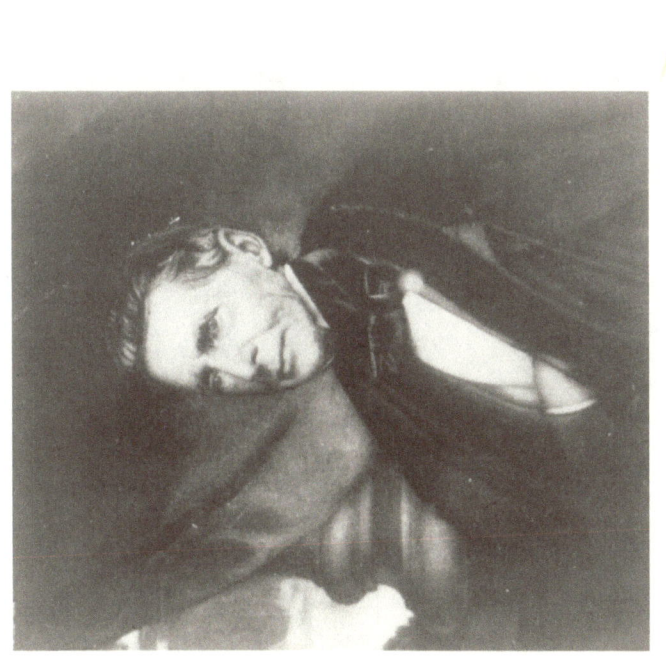

John C. Warren (1778-1856)
Courtesy Army Medical Library

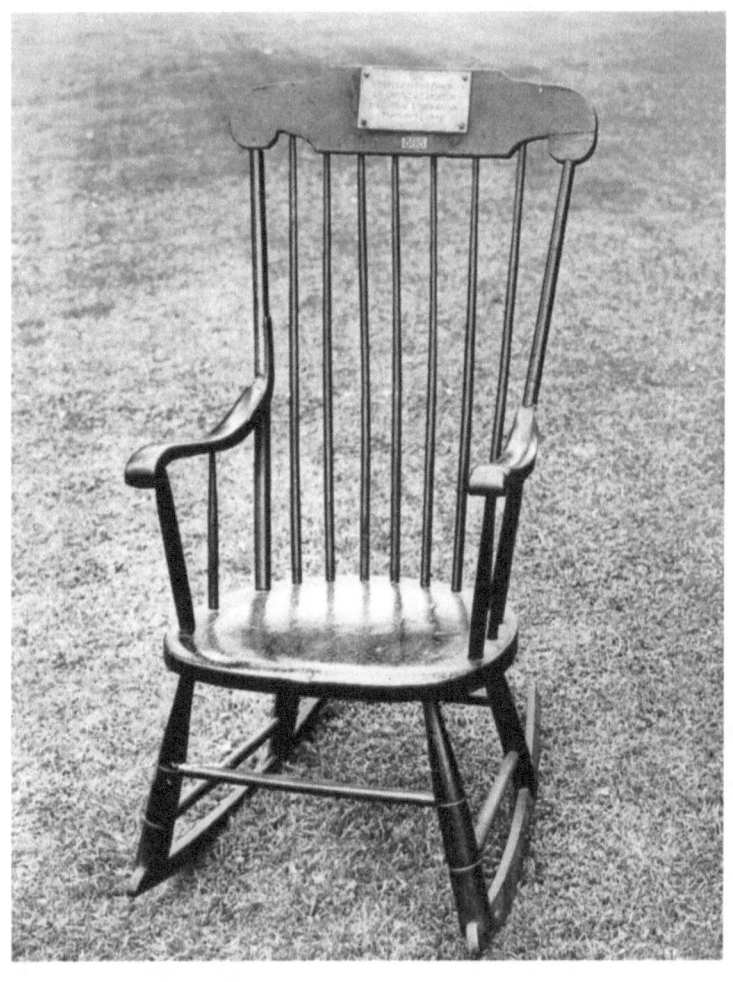

Chair in which Jackson claimed to have discovered anesthesia, "February 1842"
Photo by Randall W. Abbott, The Memorial Press

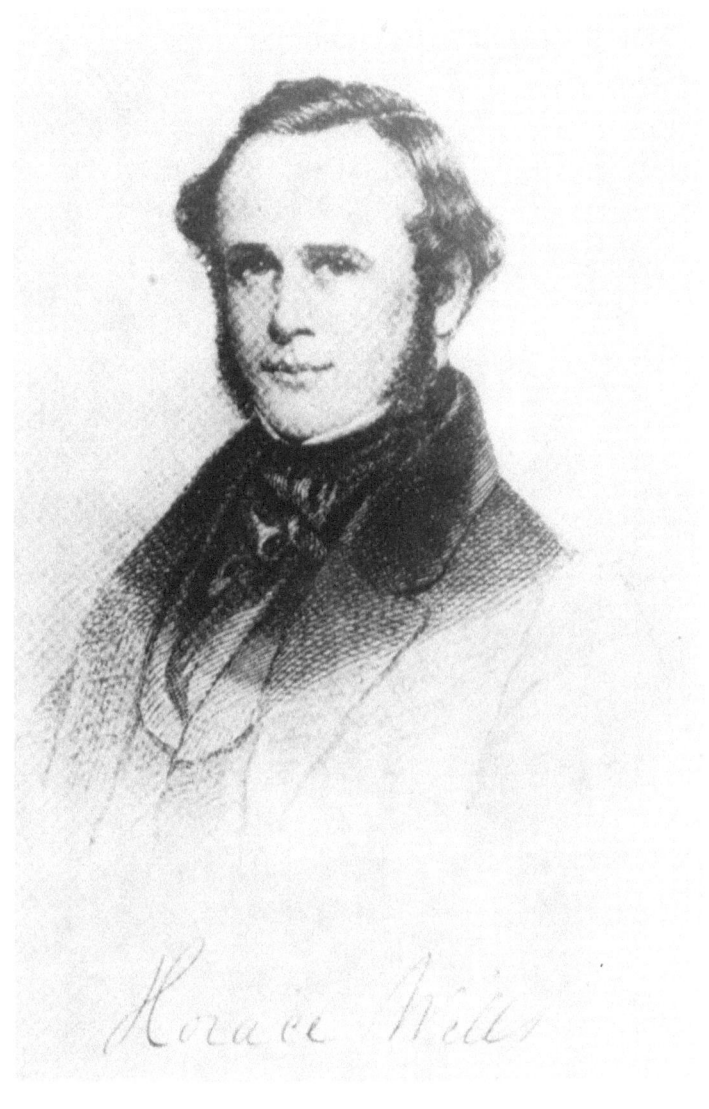

Horace Wells (1815-1848)
Courtesy Boston Medical Library

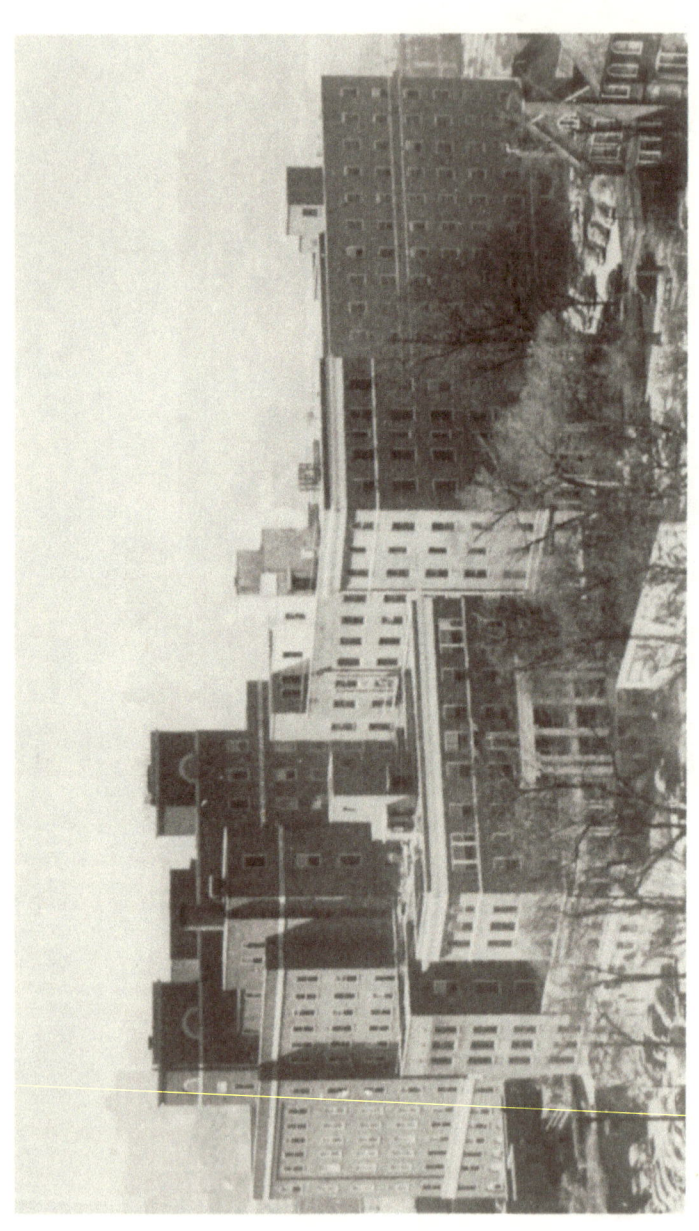

Crawford W. Long Memorial Hospital, Atlanta, Georgia

dentist, acclaimed by hosts as the discoverer of anesthesia, died in 1868, at the age of forty-eight.

JACKSON

And now to tell what we have learned about Charles Thomas Jackson, from Dr. Bunch and other sources. Dr. Jackson was born in 1805, in the historic town of Plymouth, Massachusetts. He was ten years Crawford Long's senior. We all know how young men look up to others only a few years older than themselves, and so Long looked up to Jackson. From all accounts he admired Dr. Jackson as a man and as a scientist. Jackson had an impressive educational and cultural background. It is noteworthy that his sister was the second wife of Ralph Waldo Emerson. In keeping with the custom of the times, Jackson first studied medicine under two distinguished tutors, Dr. James Jackson and Dr. Walter Channing, and graduated M.D., with honors, from Harvard, in 1829. Following this he spent three years in Europe studying medicine and geology. In Vienna he performed autopsies upon two hundred patients who had died of cholera.

But Jackson's preference was for geology and chemistry. He once said that he regretted the time he had spent studying medicine. He became prominent as a geologist, completed many important surveys, and was the first geologist of Maine, Rhode Island, and New Hampshire. It was his fondness for geology which led him into the land of Crawford Long and the gold country of Dahlonega, Georgia, fifty miles from Jefferson. He was a prodigious worker and writer. Woodworth [42] lists more than four hundred papers and discussions credited to Jackson. During a geological conference no one seemed to be better informed than he. He had a world-wide reputation as a geologist and chemist, with memberships in leading societies, but through his ambitions and the means he adopted to realize them, this man has been denounced as few men in high places have been. In his attempts to confiscate what belonged to others, however, it must be admitted that he coveted only great things, such as the invention of the telegraph, for example. But instead of adding more censure and abuse, let us recount the incidents upon which the accusations rest. So far as we know, Jackson failed in every effort to seize as his own the discoveries and inventions of others.

"JACKSON KNEW HOW TO SAVE A SECRET."

This expression appears in the Congress Reports on the Ether Controversy, and is found to be frequently applicable in the present discussion. Already described is his treatment of Morton, when, after they had agreed to claim the discovery jointly, Jackson advised the French Academy secretly that it was he who made the discovery, and failed to mention Morton's name. In 1834,[43] before this happened, Dr. Jackson had tried to appropriate from Dr. William Beaumont his human specimen, the French half-breed *voyageur*, Alexis St. Martin, whose accidental gastric fistula was enabling Beaumont to learn the physiology of the stomach to an extent never known before. When Beaumont, with the patient he was supporting for scientific investigation, was about to be removed to St. Louis, Jackson circulated a petition among the members of the Congress urging that Beaumont be sent to Boston instead. There might not have been anything wrong with this if Jackson had first informed Dr. Beaumont of what he was doing, but Surgeon General Lovell wrote that the petition was presented without the knowledge or desire of Dr. Beaumont. Beaumont had sent a specimen of St. Martin's gastric juice to Jackson, and it is believed he was intent upon performing experiments of his own and wished to keep the *voyageur* where he could reach him.

As a climax, Dr. Beaumont later received a letter, purporting to come from Alexis St. Martin, with his mark attached, saying, "I have received a letter a few months ago from a Mr. Davis Campbell, corresponding secretary of the American Physiological Society of the city of Boston, in Massachusetts, offering to engage me for a period of three to six months to be placed under the direction of an eminent physician for the purpose of experiments on digestion similar to those you have made."

Knowing the desire of the ambitious scientist to secure the invaluable St. Martin for his own, there can be but little doubt that the "eminent physician" was none other than Charles T. Jackson himself. Such an unworthy effort to further his prestige failed, like others.

On the S. S. *Sully* with Jackson, returning from his trip to Europe in 1832, was Samuel F. B. Morse,[44] a Boston artist, destined to become a great inventor. In discussing the newly discovered electro-magnet, a gentleman asked if the flow of electricity was retarded by the length of wire, whereupon Dr. Jackson said, "No, the passage of electricity through wire is instantaneous." "If this be so," added Morse, "and the presence of electricity can be made visible at any desired part of the circuit, I see no reason why intelligence might not be instantaneously transmitted to any distance."

With this idea in his head Morse returned home, and after many months of experiment perfected the telegraph and in 1837 applied for a patent. Then Jackson, with characteristic audacity, wrote Morse that he had seen notices of "our" telegraph in the papers, and demanded that he be given credit for the suggestions he had made on board the *Sully*. Receiving no encouragement from Morse, Jackson wrote again claiming that he was the principal inventor, and finally that he was "the" inventor. He was so insistent in the matter, as he had been in others like it, that a decision of the United States Supreme Court was required to declare Morse the sole inventor of the telegraph.

In addition to these three unsavory acts of Charles T. Jackson, he also contested C. F. Schonbein's[45] discovery of gun cotton in 1845,* and it is said that he claimed to have discovered the circulation of the blood, the immortal achievement of William Harvey, in 1628. I cannot find the authority for the last declaration, and feel that when it was made certainly Dr. Jackson was nearing the end of his normal mentality. This record of events in Jackson's life is well recognized by medical writers, but usually merely mentioned and passed. This the present author cannot do, because the repetition of so many incredible acts of this kind leads one to the inevitable conclusion that Jackson would commit others. If he thus attempted to seize discoveries from Morton, Morse, Beaumont and Schonbein, why would he not treat Crawford Long in a similar manner? He had the opportunity, as we shall show. *The stories of attempted confiscations herein related have been published repeatedly, and have not been denied.*

JACKSON VISITS THE MINES.

To explain why he believed "they learned about anesthesia from Crawford Long," Dr. Joseph Jacobs stated that there was unprecedented travel to and from Dahlonega,** Georgia, in the period between 1829 and 1849, on account of the gold which was being mined there. In order to reach the mining town in those days it was necessary to go by stage coach from Athens through Jefferson and Gainesville, a distance of some seventy miles. The usual

---

* Schonbein (1799-1868), of Germany, also discovered ozone.
** Dahlonega, the Cherokee Indian name for gold.

route from the East to this part of the country was to travel to Augusta, Georgia's second oldest city, and then take a coach which ran a regular route from Augusta to Dahlonega. The Georgia Railroad, the oldest in the state, began running trains from Augusta to Athens in 1841, and after that time a passenger could ride on a train to the latter town, and then go by stage coach the balance of the journey.* Jacobs said that among other stations on this hard trip, the coach stopped at Jefferson for lunch, and to water or change the horses.** This notice was found in the Georgia State Library:

The Southern Banner, May 25, 1833, announced that Banks & Longstreet opened a stage coach line running three times per week from Athens to Dahlonega, "in the heart of the gold belt;" and the Southwestern Mail Route from Washington, D. C. to New Orleans, boasted that it passed "through the Famed Gold Region of N. C. and Ga."

During the pause for refreshment at Jefferson, Dr. Jacobs visualized passengers walking around the village to stretch their legs. In so doing Jacobs suggested that a man of a scientific bent like Dr. Jackson, always on the lookout for something new and worth while, might easily have heard of the amazing occurrence which had taken place in Jefferson when a young doctor performed a surgical operation upon a patient without causing him any pain! If Jackson really first learned of successful surgical anesthesia in this manner, how the announcement must have made him prick up his ears! Then the idea would have "flashed into his

* Miss Ella May Thornton, State Librarian, furnished authentic data on the stage coach route, while Charles H. Phinizy, President of the Georgia Railroad, gave the information about the railroad.
** Miss Frances Smith, of Jefferson, in 1947, interviewed several inhabitants whose ancestors had lived there a long time, and they stated that they had always been told that the stage coach of the forties stopped at the hotel in Jefferson.

mind" that he "had made the discovery" he had "for so long a time been in quest of," as he wrote in a letter published further on.

No one can be sure just what year between 1842 and 1846 these incidents may have taken place. In spite of considerable research in Augusta, Athens, Jefferson, and Dahlonega, positive evidence has not been found that Jackson came to Georgia as early as 1846, but he stated himself that in addition to his publicized visit to Long in Athens, in 1854, when he also came to Jefferson and Dahlonega, he was in Dahlonega investigating the mines on two other occasions, in 1853 and 1858. From Jackson's interview with Long in 1854, one would not get the idea that he had ever been near Georgia before! When his geological surveys carried him to Dahlonega the year before, in 1853, the normal route of travel took him through Athens and Jefferson, but he said nothing to Dr. Long about having visited Athens previously. There was no reason this long after the ether discovery to keep secret a previous appearance in Georgia, but if he said nothing about it in 1854, why would he not fail to mention visits of other years, from 1842 to 1846, for example? In 1858 he wrote of the trip to Georgia which he made in 1853, as is shown further on.

If Dr. Jackson stopped at Jefferson any time before 1846, the year might have been 1842, very soon after Long's first experience with anesthesia, when the town was buzzing with talk of the young man's accomplishment. Always with a listening ear for a new discovery in science, Jackson, in Boston, may have heard of Long's work very soon after it happened, through agencies to be mentioned, and may or may not have undertaken the difficult journey to Georgia to investigate.

In 1857 Dr. Long wrote home from Baltimore of a trip

he was attempting to make to New York. The first day one journeyed leisurely to Augusta, where the night was spent unless one was reckless enough to travel at night. The letter read: "You will see from the heading of my letter that I have met with my usual luck and am again detained in this city for a day. This has happened to me for the three last times I have started to New York. We arrived this morning at nine o'clock and will remain until some time tonight. We missed connection at Weldon which threw us about twelve hours behind time and this detention here will make us about twenty-four to thirty hours later getting to Philadelphia than expected. We will however reach Philadelphia tomorrow in time to transact some business, if we meet with no accident. At Augusta we were advised to make the route through Columbia, S. C., and strike the Wilmington line at Weldon, N. C. The Wilmington and Manchester line, the one I have usually travelled, passes through a very swampy country, and for miles over trestles and bridges, on which several accidents have occurred lately. A detention of one night in the swamps is almost certain to produce fever." Such a trip amounted to a perilous adventure in those days.

Eighteen forty-two might be suspected as the date when Jackson first became informed of Crawford Long's success with anesthesia because Jackson, in several declarations said he *thought* it was "February, 1842" that he himself first discovered ether anesthesia, when, without any witnesses, he felt the effects of inhaling the vapor of the drug. It would seem that he could give a more exact date for such an important event as the discovery of anesthesia. Did Charles T. Jackson, with knowledge of Long's successful anesthesia of March 30, 1842, deliberately fix *his* date during the preceding month of February; or did he know nothing about

Crawford Long, and was the significant date only a coincidence?

In a letter written by Dr. Long, to be shown further on, he speaks of the possibility of Morton and Wells having visited Jefferson in 1842, but does not mention Jackson. The two men described might have been Morton and Wells, as Long suggests, but there is no other evidence to support the idea. It indicates, however, that Crawford Long, as well as others, suspected *some one* of conveying information of his anesthetic to Boston. Neither of these mysterious strangers appears to have been Dr. Jackson, although one of them easily could have been. Although he claimed to have made the great discovery in February, 1842, Jackson gave various excuses for failing to publish it to the world until 1846. He asserted that before announcing his finding he wished to give it further experimentation; and besides he was busy with his other scientific affairs. He further explained that he had retired from the medical profession, and had no facilities for research, and had no access to subjects for experiments.

Without stating that he visited Alabama, North Carolina, and Georgia during the years the articles were published, Jackson wrote frequently about the geology of these states, his first contribution appearing in the *American Journal of Science* in 1838, (xxxiv, 332-337) concerning the chemical analysis of meteoric iron from Claiborne county, Alabama, just across the Georgia line. Another article on Alabama meteoric iron was printed in the *Transactions of the American Geologists, and Naturalists*, in 1845 (207-209). Does it mean anything that Jackson's published papers, mostly on geology, appeared every year between 1832 and 1873, forty-one years, except 1842? Could he have been travelling to Georgia during that year?

The story of extensive gold-mining in the region of Dahlonega, Georgia, one hundred years ago is not well known today.* It first began in 1829 and continued with but little interruption until stopped by the California boom in 1849 and the Civil War in 1861. From 1829 to 1839 the yield was from sixteen to twenty million dollars. The government established a mint which turned out six million dollars in coin between 1838 and 1861. A writer in the *Pittsburgh Evening Telegraph* in 1876** said there were at times from ten to fifteen thousand miners at work within a radius of ten to fifteen miles of Dahlonega. No other sound arouses men like the cry of "gold." In any sort of a "gold rush," it would be easy to travel unrecognized. In the Georgia State Library and the Carnegie Library of Atlanta is found a small volume entitled, "From Report upon the Gold Placers in the vicinity of Dahlonega, Lumpkin county, Georgia, by Charles T. Jackson, M.D., Assayer to the State of Massachusetts, which were reported upon by William T. Blake, Esq., August, 1858," in which Jackson's letter starts thus:

To T. C. A. Dexter, Esq.,
 Treasurer, Yahoola River and
 Cane Creek Hydraulic Mining Co.
In accordance with your request and instructions, I left Boston on the 8th instant (Dec. 1858) and repaired to Dahlonega, Lumpkin Co., Ga. . . . Having on two previous explorations of this gold region, in 1853 and 1854, made myself pretty well acquainted with the various placers or deposits of gold. . . .

With our knowledge of Jackson's previous exploits, one

* The mines are still being worked.
** McCain, Andrew M., *History of Lumpkin County*, Stein Printing Co., Atlanta, 1932, p. 101.

cannot help but wonder if he did not come to Georgia before these dates.*

JACKSON'S ACCOUNT OF HIS VISIT TO LONG

A reproduction of this letter is appropriate at this point. It is taken from the *Boston Medical and Surgical Journal*, 64: 229-231, April 11, 1861:

The following communication is of special interest, coming as it does from one of the claimants to the exclusive credit of the introduction of sulphuric ether to the world as an anesthetic. It does not, in our opinion, invalidate in the least, the claims of either of these gentlemen, but it is of considerable importance as a matter of history. (Editorial comment).

Messrs. Editors:

At the request of Hon. Mr. Dawson, U. S. Senator from Georgia, on March 8, 1854, I called upon Dr. C. W. Long of Athens, Georgia, while on the way to the Dahlonega Gold Mines, and examined Dr. Long's evidence on which his claims to the first practical use of ether in surgical operations were founded, and wrote, as requested by Mr. Dawson, who was then in the United States Senate, all I learned on the subject.

From the documents shown me by Dr. Long, it appeared that he used sulphuric ether as an anesthetic agent:

(1) On March 30, 1842, when he excised a tumor from the neck of James Venable, a boy in Jefferson, Jackson Co., Ga., now dead.

(2) July 3, 1842, in the amputation of the toe of a negro boy belonging to Mrs. Hemphill, of Jackson Co., Ga.

(3) September 9, 1843, in the amputation of a tumor from the head of Mary Vinson, of Jefferson, Ga.

* Descendents of the family of Dr. L. D. Dugas, of Augusta, have a letter written in 1867 by Jackson to Dugas which shows that Jackson visited Dugas in Augusta in 1853. The search is being continued to learn if Dr. Jackson came to Georgia before that date.

(4) January 8, 1845, in the amputation of a finger of a negro boy belonging to Ralph Bailey, of Jackson Co., Ga.

Copies and depositions proving these operations with ether were all shown me by Dr. Long, who stated to me that his account book, with original entries and charges, was in the hands of his attorney at Jefferson, his former residence, for the purpose of having his dues collected, and that he would show me the book when I visited Athens at a future day. He also referred me to physicians in Jefferson who knew of the operations at the time. I then called on Professors Joseph and John LeConte, then of the University of Georgia at Athens, and inquired if they knew Dr. Long and what his character was for truth and veracity. They both assured me that they knew him well and that no one who knew him would doubt his word and that he was an honorable man in all respects.

Subsequently on revisiting Athens Dr. Long showed me his folio Journal, or account book, in which stand the following entries:

JAMES VENABLE

March 30, 1842—Ether and excising tumor $2.00
May 13, 1842—Sulphuric ether .... .25
June 6, 1842—Excising tumor* 2.00

On the upper half of the same page are several charges for ether sold to the teacher of the Jefferson Academy, which Dr. Long told me was used by the teacher in exhibiting its exhilarating effects, and he said the boys used it for the same purpose in the Academy. I observed that all these records bore the appearance of old and original entries in the book. Of that I have no doubt. The only question is, was the ether thus charged to Mr. Venable employed by inhalation for the purpose of preventing pain and was it actually so used in the surgical operation charged at the time?

The proof of this must be in the statement of Dr. Long

* This operation not included in Jackson's list of operations.

supported by the affidavits of the parties on whom the operations were performed or who witnessed them. These documents as above stated I have seen in the hands of Dr. Long, or rather copies of them, for the originals were sent to Dr. Paul F. Eve, of Augusta, Ga., and were lost by him, so they did not appear in the *Southern Medical Journal* then published by that gentleman.

On asking Dr. Long why he did not write to me, or make known what he had done, he said when he saw my dates I had made the discovery before him, and he did not suppose anything done after that would be considered of much importance, and that he awakened to the importance of asserting his claims to the first surgical use of ether in operations by learning that such claims were set up by others, and consequently wrote to the Georgia delegation in Congress stating the facts which Senator Dawson requested me to inquire into.

I have waited expecting Dr. Long to publish his statements and evidences in full, and have, therefore, not published what I learned from him. He is a very modest and retiring man, and not disposed to bring his claims before any but a medical or scientific tribunal. This he has done in the State Medical Society of Georgia as appears by their records. (See *Southern Medical and Surgical Journal*, Augusta, Ga.)

Had he written me in season I would have presented his claims to the Academy of Science in France, but he allowed his case to go by default, and the Academy knew no more of ether in surgical operations than I did.

(Signed) Charles T. Jackson, M.D.
Boston, April 3, 1861

Upon returning to Washington, after his visit to Georgia, Jackson gave an account of his trip to Senator Dawson, but Dr. Hugh Young[47] wrote that in a letter dated June 4, 1866, to Hon. D. L. Swain, of the University of North Carolina, Crawford Long said: "Mr. Dawson informed me that Dr. Jackson's admission of my claim was much stronger than the admission in the *Boston Medical and Surgical Journal*. He promised to furnish me with a letter of Dr. Jackson, but unfortunately soon after his health failed, and he lived but a short time." Luckily a witness was present during the meetings of Jackson and Long, Mr. C. H. Andrews, who wrote the following letter to Dr. Edwin, Newton, of Atlanta, dated at Milledgeville, Georgia, March 22, 1900. A copy of this letter was found in the Long papers. Irrelevant parts of it are omitted:

C. H. ANDREWS & SON
Insurance Agents

Dear Friend:

Recently meeting you after many years of separation and recalling incidents of our boyhood days in Athens, Ga., gave me very great pleasure. . . . You request of me a description of the old drug store in Athens, in which I served as an apprentice from August, 1849 until December, 1856, and of an interview there between Dr. Crawford W. Long and Dr. Charles T. Jackson, of Boston, Mass. . . . In 1852 C. W. and H. R. J. Long bought the drug store, and amidst the several changes I continued the principal clerk and book-keeper. The Drs. Long were brothers and both were practicing physicians.

In recalling the place where the years of my boyhood and early manhood were spent, my heart warms with gratitude and love toward my employers who were so good to me. Especially for Dr. Crawford W. Long do I cherish a reverence and love that will last to the end of my life. . . .

On March 8, 1854, early in the day, a stranger entered the store and inquired for Dr. C. W. Long. I told him Dr. Long was absent but I thought he would be in shortly, and invited him to a seat by the fireside. In a few moments Dr. Long came in, and I said, "This gentleman has called to see you." The stranger presented his card introducing himself as Dr. Charles T. Jackson, of Boston, Mass.

Dr. Jackson was a spare made man, angular, of five feet, ten inches height, of swarthy complexion, with dark eyes and hair, and apparently forty years of age. . . . Dr. Jackson said to Dr. Long that he had called to see him for the purpose of comparing notes as to the "first discovery of the anesthetic effects of sulphuric ether," they both and others claiming the discovery. Dr. Long pleasantly assented to confer with him upon the subject and I was called upon to witness their interview and to examine with them the documentary evidence each would produce.

Dr. Jackson stated that his profession was that of an analytical chemist in Boston, Mass., that a few doors from his office was the office of Dr. W. T. G. Morton, a dentist. That on September 30th, 1846, Dr. Morton came to his office and said, "Dr. Jackson, I have to perform an operation on a patient who is suffering very much and is in a very nervous condition; can you suggest or give me something that will allay pain and quiet excessive nervousness?" That he took a small vial of sulphuric ether, adding some essential oils to disguise its odor* and cautioned him in its use and fully directed him how the patient should inhale it. That the effect as an anesthetic was satisfactory and after that Dr. Morton frequently called on him for aid in that way and persevered in his efforts to learn what the article was. Finally he and Morton made a contract respecting the use of the anesthetic and applied for a patent under the name of "letheon," and in 1854 also applied to Congress for a large sum of money for the discovery. . . . That while a controversy was in progress before Congress between Jackson, Morton and Wells, it became known that Dr. Crawford W. Long had used ether in 1842, and that now he, Jackson, was there to compare notes and examine evidence as to the first discovery of ether as an anesthetic.

* Thus, Jackson not only suggested ether anesthesia to Morton, but also was responsible for disguising the odor of the drug.

Dr. Long then recited his experience with ether as an anesthetic, heretofore published, and said that during this time he conferred with physicians in all that section of Georgia, giving in detail his successful experiments and operations with sulphuric ether as an anesthetic.

[Mr. Andrews continued:] Drs. Jackson and Long submitted to my inspection much documentary proof in the way of memoranda, book entries, certificates and affidavits made under oath by patients and lookers-on. In their protracted conference they were frank but slow, cautious and exact. It was a weary day's work, and vividly before me now, though so many years intervene.

Dr. Jackson went from Athens into the gold mining region of Georgia. As he had to go through Jefferson, Ga., Dr. Long gave him names of physicians and citizens who saw and knew of his first and frequent use of ether as an anesthetic and who would personally give him their evidence.

On Dr. Jackson's return to Athens after some ten days he called upon Dr. Long again, and in my presence. Throughout their conferences during the two days that Jackson was in Athens to whatever proposition he made to Long for sharing the honor and benefits of the discovery Dr. Long replied: "My claim to the discovery of the use of sulphuric ether as an anesthetic rests upon the fact of my use of it on March 30, 1842, of which I have undisputable evidence under oath and from reputable citizens."

On taking leave of Dr. Long late in the afternoon of the second day in March, 1854, Dr. Jackson said to Dr. Long: "Well, doctor, you have the advantage of us other claimants to the first discovery of sulphuric ether as an anesthetic, but we have the advantage of having first published it to the world. . . ."

(Signed) C. H. Andrews

Georgia, Baldwin County

Personally came before me, this 15th day of November,

1900, C. H. Andrews, who being duly sworn says the statements made in the preceding letter are absolutely true.

E. P. Gibson, J.P.

In Jackson's letter concerning his visit to Long, Jackson says that Long gave as his reason for not writing him that after he saw Jackson's dates he thought Jackson had preceded him in the discovery of ether anesthesia, so that there was nothing more to be done about it. The only date to which Dr. Long could have referred was the indefinite one of "some time in February, 1842," when Dr. Jackson, without any witnesses, declared that he had felt the anesthetic effects of ether vapor, while sitting in the rocking chair. This positively did not constitute the discovery of surgical anesthesia.

From Mrs. Taylor we learn that Mr. Andrews wrote another letter in which he said: "After satisfying himself of the genuineness of the claims, Jackson proposed to Long to lay their claims conjointly before Congress: he, Jackson to claim the discovery, and Long to claim the first practical use." This proposition was rejected by Dr. Long, who was satisfied that he had discovered ether anesthesia, and also was the first to put it to practical use. The general impression has been that Jackson's object in thus approaching Crawford Long was to help defeat Morton before the Congress. I have tried to conceive a different motive, that Charles T. Jackson had an attack of *conscience*, and offered to allow Crawford Long to join with him in claiming the discovery as some compensation for failing to inform Long and the world that he had learned from him of successful surgical anesthesia.

According to Woodworth, quoted before, Dr. Jackson was State Geologist of New Hampshire from 1839 to 1843, and in 1847 began geological surveys in the region of Lake

Superior. He did not appear to hold any official position between 1843 and 1847. While engaged in geological investigations, he spent part of the time in the field and part in the laboratory. At any time he could have travelled to Georgia. He would not have visited Dahlonega as a prospector, but as an interested geologist and chemist.

Before leaving this part of the story it is well to reproduce a portion of Jackson's letter giving the grounds for his claiming to have discovered anesthesia. The statement appears in a letter addressed to Alexander Von Humboldt, and was published in Jackson's *Manual of Etherization*[48]:

The circumstances were as follows: In the winter of 1841-42 I was employed to give a few lectures before the Mechanics' Charitable Association in Boston, and in my last lecture, which I think was in the month of February, I had occasion to show a number of experiments in illustration of the theory of volcanic eruptions, and for these experiments I prepared a large quantity of chlorine gas, collecting it in gallon glass jars over boiling water. Just as one of these large jars was filled with pure chlorine, it overturned and broke, and in my endeavors to save the vessel, I accidentally got my lungs full of chlorine gas, which nearly suffocated me, so that my life was in imminent danger. I immediately had ether and ammonia brought, and alternately inhaled them with great relief. The next morning my throat was severely inflamed, and very painful, and I perceived a distinct flavor of chlorine in my breath, and my lungs were still very much oppressed.

I determined therefore to make a more thorough trial of ether vapor, and for that purpose went into my laboratory, which adjoins my house in Somerset Street, and made the experiment from which the discovery of anaesthesia was deduced. I had a large supply of perfectly pure washed sulphuric ether (oxide of ethyl), which was prepared in the laboratory of my friend, Mr. John H. Blake, of Boston.

I took a bottle of that ether and a folded towel, and having seated myself in a rocking chair, placed my feet in another chair so as to secure a fixed position as I reclined in the one in which I was seated. Soaking my towel in ether I placed it over my nose and mouth, so as to allow me to inhale the ether vapor mingled with air, and began to inhale the vapor deeply in my lungs. At first it made me cough, but soon that irritability ceased, and I noticed a sense of coolness followed by warmth, fullness of the head and chest, with giddiness and exhilaration, numbness of the feet and legs, followed by a swimming sensation as if afloat in the air. This was accompanied with entire loss of feeling, even of contact with my chair. I noticed that all sensation of pain had ceased in my throat, and the sensations which I had were of the most agreeable kind. Much pleased and excited I continued the inhalation of ether vapor, and soon fell into a dreamy state and then became unconscious of all surrounding things. I know not how long I remained in that state, but suppose that it could not have been less than a quarter of an hour, judging from the degree of dryness of the cloth which during the stage of unconsciousness had fallen from my mouth and nose, and lay upon my chest.

As I became conscious, I observed that there was no feeling of pain in my throat, and my limbs were still deeply benumbed, as if the nerves of sensation were fully paralyzed. A strange thrilling now began to be felt along the spine, but it was not in any way disagreeable. Little by little sensation began to manifest itself, first in the throat and body, and gradually it extended to the extremities; but it was some time before full sensation returned and my throat became really painful.

Reflecting on these phenomena, the idea flashed into my mind that I had made the discovery I had for so long a time been in quest of—a means of rendering the nerves of sensation temporarily insensible, so as to admit of the performance of a surgical operation on an individual without his suffering pain therefrom.

That I did draw this inference, and did fully declare my unqualified belief both of the safety and efficiency of this method of destroying all sensation of pain in the human body during the most severe surgical operations no one doubts, and it is fully proved by abundant legal evidence, which has never been impeached or doubted in any quarter.

JACKSON FROM LONG

The state of Georgia, in the eighteen-forties, with thousands of men travelling to the Dahlonega area, lent itself invitingly to hidden actions—a favorite practice of Dr. Jackson, as when he told the French Academy of Science, secretly, "I discovered anesthesia," without mentioning Morton's name; and attempted to hold Beaumont's famous Alexis St. Martin where he could experiment upon him, without consultation with Dr. Beaumont. Having learned of Crawford Long's successful anesthetic, through other possible ways to be described, Jackson journeyed to Georgia to verify what he had heard or, as has been observed, he may have learned it quite by accident as he passed through Jefferson on his way to the gold mines. In order to fit into our theory, the date of this occurrence had to be between 1842 and 1846, and the earliest year we are positive of his coming is 1853, but is that conclusive evidence that the ambitious, ingenious Jackson did not arrive before 1846?

How could he have heard away up in Massachusetts, of the master stroke of the young country doctor in remote, isolated Jefferson, Georgia? At least two other ways remain to be proposed, and the first one is found in Keys' book,[49] in which he reproduces a holograph letter of Dr. Long. Says Keys, "Its authenticity is attested by a letter written by Dr. Long's daughter, Mrs. Frances Long Taylor. Mrs.

Taylor's letter presents evidence to show that this was the first draft of a letter written to Dr. G. L. McCleskey, 'who was living near Jefferson, Ga., at the time of the visit of the two men from Boston, and who recalls the name of one who operated upon a Miss Adeline McClendon for strabismus, Dr. [Y.] Bentley. The name of the dentist he had forgotten. They remained in town a week. I think 1844 was the time he gives as the time of their visit.' " Dr. Long's letter, part of Logan Clendening's remarkable collection, reads as follows:

Permit me to say then, that a Dentist and a surgeon from Boston, Mass., were in Jefferson, Jackson County in 1842, 1843 or 1844, and remained for several weeks. The dentist practiced his profession and the surgeon operated for strabismus—I have always thought that the Dentist was Morton or Wells, & that a knowledge of my use of ether in surgical operations was obtained at that time.

I have not been able to ascertain the name of the dentist, if you know the history of Dr. Wells, you can possible ascertain whether he travelled South at the time mentioned.

This letter and the succeeding one, are only fragments, undated and unsigned. The date was sometime after 1846, otherwise he would not have known about Morton's activities. Going through Dr. Long's remaining papers in 1947 revealed an incomplete letter, in the same handwriting found in Mrs. Clendening's holograph copy, which Mrs. Taylor identified as belonging to her father. Just why Mrs. Taylor spoke of the Clendening letter as the "first draft" is not clear. Part of the writing below of Crawford Long might be the "second draft" since it gives the more definite date of 1842, instead of 1843 or 1844. People wrote and kept second copies of their letters in those days since there was no carbon paper. One reason for Long's apparent carelessness in completing and signing letters once started was his sense of duty to his patients, which we must not overlook. Caring for them always was his first consideration. On two occasions we know that he left unfinished letters, probably of historic value, to attend a woman in labor or give aid to a sick child. Sometimes these trips consumed one or two whole days.*

The first part of the letter which I found is discussing the article Jackson wrote about his visit to Georgia, suggested by Senator Dawson:

... on whom 1st operation was performed—He omits the 2nd operation, performed on the same person, J. M. Venable, on the 6th June 1842—Dr. Jackson styles J. M. V. a *boy*, probably from the fact that at the time he was a pupil in the Jackson Co. Academy. He was from 21 to 25 years old, as were a large number of the pupils at that time in the academy. 3rd operation (Dr. Jackson's 2nd) correct.

Most of the depositions and letters obtained were procured to establish these operations. The evidence to establish the operation after 1842 were only obtained to shew that the operations were certain up to the time of Dr. Wells claims to have made the discovery. Permit me to say here that I have had a strong belief, that Dr. Wells or Morton, were in Jefferson, Jackson Co., Ga., in 1842 or there, while there was much talk of my operations & obtained the Knowledge of Anesthetic properties of Ether at that time—

In one of these years there was a Dentist and an operator

* William Guy Minder, of Atlanta, is the author of an entertaining account of Long and his discovery of anesthesia, used as script for radio performances. As confirming Long's adherence to what he considered his duty, Minder relates the authentic story that Dr. Long was so late arriving for his wedding to Caroline Swain, in 1842, that many of the guests took their departure, to avoid the embarrassment of witnessing the failure of the bridegroom to "show up." He did arrive, however, and explained that he had been detained by a very sick patient. Soon after the ceremony he told Caroline that he must go back to the patient, which he did, not returning to his bride until the following morning.

for deformities and diseases of the eye, from Boston. Their names I have been unable to obtain.

Mrs. Taylor's explanation of the first letter mentions names which investigation showed might offer ways for Jackson to know of Long's successful surgical anesthetic. In this, invaluable aid was given by those named in "Acknowledgements." Dr. G. L. McCleskey, to whom Dr. Long wrote the letter, married Georgiana Bird Washburn in 1841, at the home of her aunt, Mrs. Lamar, afterwards Mrs. Troutman, in Oxford, Georgia. Mrs. Lamar was the mother of the celebrated L. Q. C. Lamar, United States Senator from Mississippi. It is interesting that Mrs. McClesky, although born in Georgia, was descended from the prominent Washburn family in Massachusetts, some of whom lived in Bridgewater, Leicester, and other places. Among these was Emory Washburn, Governor of Massachusetts, 1854-55. Mrs. McCleskey's father, Joseph Washburn, although later a successful banker of Savannah, Georgia, was born in Bridgewater, Massachusetts, and it is again interesting, although possibly not significant, that the town of Bridgewater is located in Plymouth county, the county of historic Plymouth by the sea, the birthplace of Charles T. Jackson. Bridgewater lies about fifteen miles west of Plymouth and on the way to Boston, although it is not certain that in traveling from Plymouth to Boston in the 1840's one would pass through Bridgewater.

We may be going out of the way slightly to build up Dr. Jackson's chances for deceit, but the case calls for imagination to match his methods. The writer again affirms that he has no desire to cast aspersions on anyone's character. The whole motive is to present Long as the discoverer, the originator, of surgical anesthesia; Jackson as the messenger to Morton; and Morton as the public demonstrator of medicine's greatest gift to humanity, always remembering the role played by the Boston surgeons. If this sequence of events is correct, Crawford Long's contribution entitles him to be numbered among those who introduced surgical anesthesia to the world.

That Dr. Long should write this letter to Dr. McCleskey would indicate that they were close friends. What would be more natural, then, that young Mrs. McCleskey, just married, in 1841, in corresponding with some of her relatives in Bridgewater, and other places in Massachusetts, would mention the remarkable feat of her husband's friend, another doctor, Crawford Long? Such news could be understood by laymen, and they would spread it. If the announcement had been that Claude Bernard had discovered the vaso-motor nerves, or had described the glycogenic function of the liver, that would have been too technical for lay people to appreciate or talk about. But finding a way of performing a surgical operation without pain would be a matter of public interest and a discovery which would impress intelligent laymen. They would discuss it and write about it. Today it would be front-page news in big type. Also, it is recorded that Mrs. McCleskey attended school in Philadelphia, and she may have made friends of some young women of Massachusetts with whom she corresponded. Research has failed to reveal any letters of Mrs. McCleskey, but it must be remembered that people wrote more letters, and longer letters, one hundred years ago than they do today. If intelligence of Long's discovery reached Bridgewater, the ever wide-awake and receptive Jackson, in Plymouth or Boston, could easily have heard of it. Woodworth[50] says Jackson addressed the Plymouth County Agricultural Society, in Bridgewater, September 25, 1850, and goodness knows how many times he had been there before.

To verify another name mentioned in Mrs. Taylor's explanatory letter, Miss Frances Smith writes of an elderly lady who stated that she had heard her mother speak of Miss Adeline McClendon, of the 1840's, and had visited in her home. Dr. [Y.] Bentley, also mentioned in the letter, cannot be identified. The Massachusetts Medical Society has no record of such a member.

Jackson Knew it Would Work

The extreme confidence with which Dr. Jackson assured Morton of the practicability and safety of ether anesthesia is most significant. The *Congress Reports* reveal several instances which show that Jackson had positive information that successful surgical anesthesia was a fact. How could he be so sure of this unless he had knowledge that the long waited-for event had occurred? He could not know it from the mere suggestions of Humphry Davy, nor from the experiment which he claimed to have done on himself. To Dr. George T. Dexter, in 1842, he declared in the *Congress Reports*, ether anesthesia "to be a safe and efficient means of preventing all sensations of pain in all surgical operations, and spoke freely, *earnestly and confidently* of the discovery as a means of alleviating much human suffering." In a letter to Jackson, in the same *Reports*, Henry Sumner wrote:

"Calling at your office a day or two after you had communicated your discovery to Mr. Morton, of the use of sulphuric ether as an agent for destroying pain in the extraction of teeth, I distinctly recollect hearing you affirm with *great confidence and enthusiasm* that the severest *surgical operations* could be performed upon patients under the influence of that agent, without giving them the slightest pain."

In a letter from Dr. William F. Channing, of Boston, a Fellow of the American Academy of Arts and Sciences appears: "I have heard Dr. Jackson speak on several occasions of the inhalation of sulphuric ether for producing insensibility to pain during operations of a surgical nature. These conversations with Dr. Jackson took place, according to my recollection, during the summer or autumn of 1842."

In the year 1846, and before the 30th of September, Henry D. Fowle, a Boston druggist, in an affidavit affirmed: "Dr. Jackson then again spoke with *perfect confidence* of the power of the ethereal vapor to destroy the pain of surgical operations."

D. Jay Browne, of New York, wrote in a letter to Jackson, "You spoke with *great enthusiasm* and *earnestness* of this discovery [Jackson's], stating that the means proposed by you was both efficient and safe, and would prevent any sensation of pain, even in the most severe surgical operations."

No one had ever before spoken with such absolute conviction of the practicability of surgical anesthesia. Indeed, no one at this time was qualified so to speak except Crawford Long. There is no record that Dr. Jackson was ever asked how he *knew* surgical anesthesia was a success, when his whole personal experience consisted in rendering himself unconscious in a rocking chair, without witnesses. Granting his report of this incident was true, that did not constitute surgical anesthesia. Surgical anesthesia means an actual successful surgical operation upon a patient, without pain. The positive assurance he expressed leads to no other conclusion than that Jackson knew of at least one operation in which ether had been safely and satisfactorily employed as an anesthetic, and who could have done this at this time except Crawford Long? That Jackson told some of these witnesses in 1842 of his positive confidence in surgical anesthesia would indicate that he learned of Long's success in that year.

Jackson to Morton

As recorded in the Congress Reports on the Ether Discovery, 1852-1863, Jackson testified, and several witnesses heard him, that when he suggested ether anesthesia to Morton, the young dentist said, "Ether? What is it?" But Morton explained later that this was only an evasive answer. He added that he knew what ether was, because he had experimented with it; but he wished to keep Jackson in ignorance of his knowledge of the substance and its properties, because he was planning to introduce it as an anesthetic, and expected to make a great deal of money from it, in which he did not care for Jackson to share. One may believe Morton's story or not, but the whole account of the controversy does not substantiate it. Most authors speak of the incident without comment, but Raper,[51] who supports Morton's claims as the discoverer, is not convinced that Morton performed any of the experiments which he mentioned.

Raper says: "Of the six experiments Morton claimed he made on himself and his assistants, it is doubtful if he made any, with the possible exception of the one on himself on September 30th, the same day he gave ether to Eben Frost."

In spite of the dentist's protestations to the contrary, most recent writers on the history of anesthesia believe that Morton obtained the knowledge of the practical use and safety of ether anesthesia from Dr. Jackson. Otherwise why should Morton have agreed to allow Jackson to share the patent with him, and upon Jackson's withdrawing his name as a patentee, why should Morton grant Jackson ten per cent of the profits?

Victor Robinson[52] writes, "Jackson suggested to Morton that he use ether in extracting a tooth."

Fulton[53] says, "September 30th, 1846, Jackson suggested

that he use ether inhalation to pull Eben Frost's tooth."

Keys[54] is not so positive. In his book we read, "Jackson recommended that he try pure sulfuric ether. Morton professed ignorance of the use of sulfuric ether, and Jackson later based his claim to the discovery on his suggestion to Morton that ether would anesthetize the patient. Morton did find out from Jackson, however, that pure sulfuric ether would serve his purpose better than the commercial product."

In the *Congress Reports*, Morton is called the "great pretender": he *pretended* to Jackson that the use of ether as an inhalent anesthetic was new to him, just as he *pretended* that he had added aromatic oils to ether to make it a more efficient agent, whereas the information was later extracted from him that the foreign ingredients were added to disguise the chief substance, ether ("letheon").

In Garrison's classical work[55] is read, "Morton learned from Jackson that sulphuric ether is also an anesthetic," while Castiglioni[56] declares that ether was suggested to Morton by the chemist, Dr. C. T. Jackson.

Haggard[57] writes, "One of his professors, a chemist named Jackson, suggested to him that he try ether instead of gas."

Lambert and Goodwin[58] say, "Morton undertook some experiments on animals with ether at the suggestion of Dr. Jackson."

The *Encyclopedia Britannica*, Fourteenth Edition, sums the matter up well when it affirms, "On Sept. 30, 1846, Dr. W. T. G. Morton, a dentist of Boston, following the suggestion of Dr. C. T. Jackson, employed the vapour of ether in private to procure general anesthesia in a case of tooth extraction, and thereafter administered it in cases requiring surgical operation with complete success."

In his text-book on surgery Dr. John Homans,[59] grandson of another John Homans, whose name appears in the Ether Controversy, writes, "He (Morton) is said to have known the intoxicating quality of ether as a student in 1839, but in any case he obtained a full knowledge of ether's qualities from Dr. Charles T. Jackson, an experienced chemist."

Witnesses under oath, in the *Congress Reports*, were even more positive that Morton was indebted to Jackson for his knowledge of ether anesthesia as applied to surgery. These witnesses, relying upon Morton's testimony, gave Jackson credit for the discovery.

Said D. P. Wilson, of Boston: "Respecting the authorship of the discovery, I do not feel the least embarrassment or doubt; for my opinion has been wholly founded upon the narrative and declarations of Mr. Morton, in which, uniformly and without reserve, he ascribed its authorship to Dr. Jackson, never speaking of himself otherwise than as the first and fortunate person to whom Dr. Jackson had communicated it."

Said Alvah Blaisdell, of Boston: "At that time—on or about the last of September or the first of October—I had a conversation with Dr. Morton to the following effect: I asked him how he succeeded in the application of ether. He replied, 'Most satisfactorily.' I then asked him how he had dared to use an agent so powerful. He told me that he had received the most positive assurance from Dr. C. T. Jackson, that it was perfectly safe. I remarked, 'then you have consulted Dr. Jackson?' He replied in the affirmative, and stated that the idea of employing sulphuric ether was first suggested to him by Dr. Jackson. I asked him thereupon if it was Dr. Jackson who made the discovery. Mr. Morton at once answered, 'that he did, and that Dr. Jackson had communicated it to him, with instructions as to the proper mode of applying the ether; and that having acted in accordance with his advice, his (Morton's) practice had been successful, the result in every way answering to Dr. Jackson's predictions.'"

J. A. Robinson, of Salem: "Morton unreservedly admitted that there was someone behind himself connected with the discovery as its originator, and that person was Dr. Charles T. Jackson."

Nathan B. Chamberlain, Boston: "Mr. Morton, by his conversation, gave me every reason to believe that someone other than himself was the discoverer of the 'preparation.' He said distinctly, that it was the suggestion of another, and from Mr. Morton's manner of speaking of Dr. Jackson in connection with the 'preparation,' as he did quite frequently during the interview, no doubt was left in my mind that Dr. Jackson was the discoverer."

Horace J. Payne, Troy, New York: "Dr. Morton stated repeatedly and emphatically, that Dr. Charles T. Jackson, of Boston, was the sole discoverer of the new agent for producing insensibility to pain, and that Dr. Jackson had communicated it to him."

As declared in the *Congress Reports*, "all the witnesses are men of mature age, and none of them have been discredited." Other depositions of similar emphatic, clear language were published, and could be reproduced, but these, taken with the statements of authors of recent books, seem sufficient to confirm the fact that Morton learned of the feasibility and safety of surgical anesthesia from Charles T. Jackson.

8

AFTERWARDS

IN 1850, DESIRING A LARGER location for his growing practice, Dr. Long, with his family, moved to the new city of Atlanta, about eighty miles from Jefferson. Five years previously John C. Calhoun had predicted that Atlanta some day would become a great city, and signs of fulfillment were beginning to show. At this time, however, its recent growth was too evident, and Atlanta did not strike the physician as the best place in which to rear and educate children. So, after a year's residence, the Longs moved to Athens, seat of the state University, and known as the "Classic City." There were then three children living, the oldest, a son, having died. Dr. and Mrs. Long had twelve children, three sons and nine daughters, but only seven of the number lived to maturity. The home which Crawford Long erected in Atlanta* on the southwest corner of Broad and Luckie streets, was a remarkable specimen of architecture for the middle of the nine-

---

* According to James Walter Mason, Atlanta title lawyer, Long paid Reuben Cone $350.00 for the lot, which fronted 100 feet on the present Broad street, and ran back 200 feet to Forsyth street.

teenth century. It looked as if it belonged to the present day. His residence in Athens, where he was living at the time of his death, also was an impressive structure.

The succeeding decade was a happy and prosperous one for the family. Then came rumblings of the inevitable conflict between the North and the South. Long, conforming with the position taken by his former roommate, Alexander H. Stephens, at first opposed secession and made a speech against it. But when Georgia withdrew from the Union, the two friends sided with their state. Dr. Long regarded slavery as "God's method of caring for the Negro," and looked upon the possession of his servants as a trust to be administered as a divinely imposed duty. He cared for them as members of his own family. It may not be generally known that there were slave holders in the North as well as in the South.

Mrs. Taylor did not write that her father volunteered for service in the Confederate army, but rather that "he was without solicitation, designated to remain at home as physician for the families of the soldiers, and for the wounded who had been sent home to recuperate." But now comes to light interesting information. A letter from Miss Lillian Henderson, Director of the Georgia Department of Confederate Pensions and Records, dated December 17, 1947, states that "Crawford Long enlisted from Clarke county, Georgia, as a private in Captain Taylor's Company of Georgia Infantry, July 19, 1864." He was then forty-nine years old. There is no record of his having been called to active duty, but at least he offered his services by enlisting. Dr. Long's family received a Cross of Honor from the Daughters of the Confederacy for his services, and a chapter of the organization in Atlanta bears his name. In 1867 Surgeon General J. S. Billings, of the United States Army, appointed Long surgeon at the post in Athens, which position he filled until civil government was restored. In this capacity he cared for soldiers of both armies.

A noteworthy incident occurred in 1864, so far as the discovery of surgical anesthesia is concerned. The story comes from Mrs. Taylor and Mr. Minder, and has to do with the flight which Mrs. Taylor made upon hearing that a division of Federal Cavalry was approaching Athens. The news was brought by a wounded young captain who reported that the division had orders to burn the city, take all the mules and horses, destroy all provisions, and decoy away all the Negro slaves, both male and female. Upon receiving this information at the military hospital, Dr. Long treated the officer's wound and asked him to take a note to his family at home. The message was for Frances Long, the eldest daughter (the future Mrs. Taylor), and her young brother to put the silver and other valuables in a carriage and drive to the home of the wounded captain, which was off the route of the probable march of the Federal cavalry. The coachman was ordered to hide the remaining horses in a swamp.

In the meantime Dr. Long reached home, and just as the two young people were leaving, he ran down the road with a glass jar in his hand which contained two huge gold watches and a roll of papers. He told Frances that these papers were most important and must not be lost; they were proofs of his discovery of anesthesia. "Promise me that when you reach the captain's house you will bury the papers in a secluded spot. If overtaken by the raiders you may be frightened into giving them the jar if ordered to do so." Mrs. Taylor wrote that this speech put her on her mettle, and she replied, "I will die before I do." Arriving at her destination, Frances found the house already packed with the property of the entire community, but the captain's sister devised a plan for hiding the jar. She helped Frances lengthen her dress down to her ankles, under which she concealed the jar with a cord. When they arrived deep in the woods her companion produced a spade from under her dress and dug a hole in which they deposited the jar with its precious contents and covered the place with sticks and leaves. The next day word was received that the enemy raiders had been captured by Colonel Breckenridge at Jug Tavern, twenty miles from Athens, and the girls returned to the spot where they had buried the jar and recovered it.

From time to time we hear that Crawford Long "died in poverty and obscurity." The least effort to learn the facts concerning the life of Dr. Long would at once convince any unbiased mind of the falsity of such reports. The declaration of one writer that during his later life Long returned to the surgery of pre-anesthetic days is absolutely refuted by the history we have given. Long is also placed in the category of other claimants to the discovery as dying a tragic death.* None of the untrue statements which have been made would affect Dr. Long's status as the discoverer of anesthesia, but why not keep the record straight? Data has been given in previous chapters to show that Long continued to employ ether anesthesia in surgical operations as long as he lived. Not only was this the case in his own practice, but he was called frequently to administer ether for other doctors. As to his dying in poverty, the story of his life proves that his financial success was far above the average of practitioners of his period. He inherited property, and through an extensive practice and careful

---

* Wells committed suicide, while the true cause of Morton's death was not determined, but was believed to be due to some kind of "stroke," as a result of his long fight in Congress, the bitter disappointment in failing to obtain universal recognition, and worry over financial matters.

business methods he was able to live comfortably and care for his large family. It is true the War caused serious losses, as it did for Southern people generally, but during the twenty-three years he lived after 1865 his former financial status was largely restored. This was aided by returns from the retail and wholesale drug business conducted during this time by Dr. Long and his brother. Wells and Morton met untimely deaths, while Jackson became insane but lived to be seventy-five years of age. These sad terminations have been ascribed as partly due to the ether controversy. No such factor was present in the passing of Crawford Long, at the age of sixty-three. He was not concerned with the historical controversy as it affected the others, and if he had been, his serene disposition would have saved him from similar suffering and despair.

The following letter recently found among Dr. Long's papers, in his handwriting, throws some light upon the cause of his death. The letter was dated Feb. 2nd, 1877, sixteen months before he died, and was addressed to Dr. J. Marion Sims:

Yours of the 29th ult. has just been received, and I regret that my apparent neglect in furnishing you with the facts of my personal history, has been a source of annoyance to you. When you fully understand the real cause of the apparent neglect, you will not blame me, but regret that any such cause existed. Since I received your first note I have been a great sufferer with my head, scarcely any ease except the few days 1 was suffering so severely from the injury I received the last week in Decbr. All mental exertion increased the pain so much, that I dreaded, I might add, almost feared to make any effort. My practice which I was compelled to attend to was more than I felt myself able to accomplish. I occasionally had short periods of ease, but never felt so much confidence or hope of permanent relief as

I have felt for two days past. Although fatigued from professional engagements, I have scarcely felt a pang for the two days, and my sanguine character leads me almost to exclaim, "I am myself again." Should I suffer so again, can you suggest suitable remedy? For week past have been using mercurials, with great apparent benefit. . . .

There is nothing to show whether this letter is a copy of one which was sent to Dr. Sims, or was the copy intended for him, and never sent. Today we would diagnose Long's case as one of high blood pressure, a common condition even today in physicians of this age who have led a strenuous life.

Recognition

After following the busy, normal life of a practitioner of medicine for nearly forty years, Crawford Long came to his death suddenly, June 16, 1878. It was fitting that he should die as he had lived, "in harness," as he delivered the wife of Congressman H. H. Carlton. His last articulate words were, "Care for the mother and child first." The cause of his death was given as cerebral hemorrhage.

Long did not die in obscurity. Extracts from the funeral oration of Dr. A. A. Lipscomb, past chancellor of the University of Georgia, show the high regard and affection in which he was held by the citizens of his home town:

"For nearly forty years he practiced medicine, with what skill, with what constancy of interest and sustained force of sympathy, with what calm enthusiasm of devotion, I need not tell you, whose homes this day are in mourning over a bereavement which is personal no less than professional to so many citizens of Athens and its vicinity. . . . 'I believe', said Dr. Long, 'that my profession is a ministry of God to me,' and again, speaking of his discovery of anesthesia, by means of sulphuric ether: 'My only wish is to be known as a benefactor of my race. . . .' Standing here in the presence of his remains, I am this day but the voice of the church, of his professional brethren, and of this whole community, when I say that in Dr. Long's death we have lost an excellent man."

A tribute of respect signed July 6, 1878, by his colleagues in Athens, read:

"Dr. Long was an honor to the profession, regarding it as a medium through which to make his life a blessing to the world. He was a high-minded Christian gentleman; always just and liberal toward his professional brethren, holding sacred their reputation as his own, by strictly observing the highest code of medical ethics in all his associations with them. He was never heard to make reflections or criticisms detrimental to any with whom he was called in consultation. As such all his neighboring practitioners held him in their highest esteem and confidence and almost invariably Dr. Long was called on to attend the sick chamber of physicians and their families. Truly did he subordinate his desire for fortune or fame, to the one great purpose of benefiting his race. His highest ambition was to do good and leave the world better by his labors. Truth, honesty and candor marked his character, while he cultivated the noble qualities of love and mercy. Not only did he visit the homes of wealth and luxury when called to relieve affliction, but was liberal in bestowing his benefactions to the poor, by carrying relief and comfort to the inmates of hovels, with no hope of reward but gratitude and love.

"Resolved, That his professional brethren do most heartily endorse the claim of Dr. C. W. Long as the first discoverer of anesthesia by the use of sulphuric ether.

"Resolved, That the highest honors are due his memory for his discovery, by which so much pain and suffering have been spared, and that we will ever regard him as a true philanthropist and benefactor of mankind.

G. L. McCleskey, M.D.
John Gerdine, M.D.
Wm. King, M.D.

R. M. Smith, M.D.
J. E. Pope, M.D.
J. B. Carlton, M.D.

Three of the most important papers written about Crawford Long were those of Marion Sims, in 1877; Luther B. Grandy, in 1893; and Hugh H. Young, in 1897, to which reference already has been made. In 1925 Leake[60] wrote: "Much has been made over the fact that Long did not publish his discovery in 1842. Morton did not publish his until 1850." It was H. J. Bigelow who announced Morton's anesthetic in 1846. Although Dr. Long put his story in print as far back as 1849, it received but little publicity, and it was not until the appearance of Dr. Sims' article, almost thirty years later, that information concerning Dr. Long's contribution to surgical anesthesia began to reach the country generally. The division of the United States by the Civil War, which occurred during this period, doubtless was a factor in retarding the broadcasting of the news of the first anesthetic.

A crayon portrait of Long, made at the time of his first anesthetic, by an unknown artist, is his earliest likeness. Following this a life-size oil painting was made by Frank G. Carpenter and presented to the State of Georgia during the meeting of the Legislature, August 22, 1879. Senator John B. Gordon made the presentation. The donor was Mr. Henry L. Stuart, a prominent citizen of New York, and a friend of Marion Sims, who had been greatly impressed by the achievement of Long. The picture, which was painted from especially made photographs, still hangs in the State Capitol. Mr. Stuart accompanied the portrait to Atlanta, after which he visited the grave of Crawford Long in Athens. Here occurred a distressing incident. Stuart became paralyzed and died after an illness of three weeks. At his request he was buried by the side of Dr. Long in Oconee Cemetery.

During the same year, 1879, Alexander H. Stephens, congressman, and former vice-president of the Southern Confederacy, in paying tribute to his old friend and roommate, Crawford Long, before the alumni of the University of Georgia, appealed to his audience to recommend that the State Legislature petition Congress to accept statues of Dr. Long and General James Oglethorpe to be placed in the House of Representatives at Washington. The suggestion was adopted, but the Legislature finally selected Dr. Long and Mr. Stephens himself for the distinction.

The Georgia physician has continued to be honored in various ways in the South and the North and in different parts of the world. Most of his citations have declared him to be the discoverer of anesthesia. To perpetuate his name and achievement, resolutions have been passed, addresses have been made, paintings unveiled, and monuments and statues erected.

The National Eclectic Medical Association, at its meeting in Cleveland, Ohio, June 18, 1879, passed a resolution expressing "its appreciation and recognition of the inestimable services which Crawford Long had rendered to medical science and humanity, as the discoverer of anesthesia."

In 1902, two prominent physicians of Mexico, David Cerna and Ramon E. Trevino, made enthusiastic addresses giving Long credit as the real discoverer.

When King Edward VII of England, in 1902, awoke from the anesthetic which had been administered to him in performing an operation for "perityphlitis," he asked his surgeon, Sir Frederick Treves, "Who discovered anesthesia?" Sir Frederick answered at once, "It was an American, your Majesty, Crawford W. Long."

Dr. George Foy, of Dublin, Ireland, a medical historian of note, espoused the cause of Crawford Long in the eighteen-eighties. In June, 1910, Dr. Foy wrote Mrs. Taylor for permission for Sir Frederick Hewett, the anesthetist for King George V, to exhibit Dr. Long's papers at a medical meeting to be held in London, where representatives from all the British possessions, including India and Australia, would be in attendance. Mrs. Taylor and her sister, Miss Emma Long, crossed the Atlantic with the yellowed papers which were put on exhibition in the British Medical Museum. Dr. Dudley W. Buxton, eminent anesthetist, after examining the documents, contributed a paper entitled, "Crawford Williamson Long, the Pioneer of Anesthesia and the First to Suggest and Employ Ether Inhalation in Surgical Operations."* Dr. Foy later wrote the following letter to a Georgia physician:

"I hunted up authorities in the British Museum Library and finally produced my book in 1886, and today, Dec. 24, 1910, I am thankful to say that Dr. C. W. Long is acknowledged as the discoverer by every one of our anaesthetists in Great Britain and my arguments in his favor have been translated into all the principal languages in Europe. Of one great fact I am sure, to wit: the principal anaesthetists of London recognize his claim to the discovery of anaesthesia as well founded and in their hospital classes they so inform their students. Dr. Long's portrait occupies an honorable place in the rooms of the Royal Society of Medicine and will hold a similar position in the new building the Society is erecting by Trafalgar Square at the cost of 30,000 pounds sterling. No writing or talking can now in London affect his position. It has been accepted and acknowledged by writers and teachers."

In April, 1910, during a meeting of the Medical As-

* Proceedings Royal Society of Medicine, 5:19-45, 1912.

sociation of Georgia, in Athens, a granite monument was dedicated to Long in Jefferson, Georgia, the scene of the first anesthetic. The memorial was the gift of Dr. Lamartine G. Hardman, of Commerce, Georgia, to the Jackson County Medical Society. In the course of his remarks as orator of the occasion, Dr. Woods Hutchinson said:

"I am here to say that wherever men speak of the achievements of science an allusion is made to the greatest boon ever made to suffering humanity—anesthesia. Dr. Crawford Long's discovery was no accident. His real genius and the proof of his greatness lay in his wisdom to see the possibilities, the courage to attempt the experiments, the confidence in his own opinions, and in the heart-felt love and sympathy for his suffering patients, which led him to employ the anesthetic which he had discovered, not once but many times. He was great in his courage, braving the possibility of the fearful consequences which would have followed in those early days of experiment. He was great in his love for his profession and affectionate sympathy for his patients. He was great in the breadth of his intellect, the culture of his mind, his familiarity and appreciation of letters and art and refinement. He was great in his services to his fellowman."

On March 30th, 1912 the seventieth anniversary of the first use of ether as an anesthetic in surgery, there was unveiled at the University of Pennsylvania a bronze medallion to Crawford W. Long, of the Class of 1839, from his alma mater. The handsome piece was the conception of the well-known sculptor, R. Tait McKenzie. Among the speakers was Dr. J. William White, of the University, whose address began as follows:

"We have come here today to do honor to the memory of a son of Pennsylvania who was the pioneer, who actually led the world in what was perhaps the most momentous attack upon pain and suffering, and indirectly upon disease itself, ever made in the history of mankind."

Dr. John Chalmers DaCosta, representing the Jefferson Medical College, thus spoke:

"Now and then a real leader, an original force, a truly great man comes into the world, and moves us as one inspired. He dares to lift the veil which hangs before the mysteries, the veil which lesser men are too ignorant to observe, too indifferent to regard, or too cowardly or incapable to displace. Such a man seeks truth and scorns wealth—courts labor and forgets ease—fights dragons and slays giants, is the slave to duty, is contemptuous of popularity, and finally wrings
'the secret of deliverance
Whether it lurk in hells or hide in heavens.'
He originates. 'Every institution,' says Emerson, 'was once the act of a single man.' "

On June 14th, 1921, the occasion of the 121st commencement exercises of the University of Georgia, a replica of McKenzie's medallion was unveiled on the campus, the gift of Crawford Long's former employee, Dr. Joseph Jacobs.

During the meeting of the Southern Medical Association in Hot Springs, Arkansas, November 16, 1921, a resolution was adopted declaring Long to be entitled to the credit and honor of the discovery of anesthesia.

A statue of Dr. Long, designed by the New York sculptor, J. Massey Rhind, and carved from Georgia marble by James K. Watt, was unveiled in Statuary Hall in the national capitol, March 30th, 1926. It is a good likeness, copied from the small crayon profile drawing, which had been made at the time of the discovery.

On April 15th, 1926, a granite boulder was dedicated

to Dr. Long in the court house yard of his birthplace, Danielsville, Georgia.

In the same year an oil painting of Long, the work of Lewis Gregg, was hung in Alumni Hall, at the University of Georgia. This portrait showed the physician at the age of twenty-six, when he gave the first anesthetic, and is an artistic triumph.* Other portraits represent Long at a later period in his life.

Dr. E. C. Davis, of Atlanta, was always a firm supporter of Crawford Long's claim to be recognized as the discoverer of surgical anesthesia. Upon the death of Dr. Davis, his partner, Dr. L. C. Fischer, in 1930, changed the name of the Davis-Fischer Sanatorium to the Crawford W. Long Memorial Hospital. Recent additions have given the institution a capacity of five hundred patients. Dr. Fischer has deeded the hospital to Emory University.

A reproduction of the marble statue in Washington was unveiled in Danielsville in 1936. Dr. Hugh H. Young was the principal speaker.

In 1934 the Fellows of the American College of Surgeons in Georgia accepted the invitation of the College to present a bronze plaque of Dr. Long to be hung in the auditorium of the John B. Murphy Memorial in Chicago.

The same year a plaque of Long was accepted by the University of Edinburgh from the Southern Society of Clinical Surgeons.

In 1940, a commemorative postage stamp was issued in honor of Dr. Long.

On the 30th of March each year the University of Georgia celebrates "Crawford Long Day," when distinguished members of the medical profession are invited to

* March 30th, 1949, the 107th anniversary of Long's discovery, a copy of this painting by Mr. Gregg, was hung in the Academy of Medicine, home of the Fulton County Medical Society, as the gift of Dr. T. J. Collier, pioneer anesthetist of Georgia.

make addresses. Among those who have accepted the invitation are Dr. Hugh H. Young, Dr. Alfred Blalock, Dr. John S. Lundy and Dr. Max Cutler.

Endorsements of Crawford Long as the discoverer of anesthesia from authoritative sources could be quoted almost without end. Many of these appear in the book and articles listed under "Bibliography." An interesting extract comes from a letter written by Dr. J. A. Redfearn, of Albany, Georgia, formerly president of the Medical Association of Georgia:

"In 1926 I stepped from the ranks of one hundred doctors from all over the nation taking Dr. Cabot's course on cardiology, after he had led us up winding stairs to the amphitheater where he reminded us in well chosen words that Dr. Morton first administered ether here. I asked to make a statement which was granted. I said that reliable records showed that Crawford Long, of Georgia, used ether in a surgical operation four years before Morton. Dr. R. C. Cabot remarked, 'Long's claim is a just claim.' Some of the doctors in the group, from different parts of the country, came to me the next day and said they did not believe my statement until they visited the Boston City Library and looked it up."

The Scotch author, Guthrie,[61] affirms, "Some writers have constructed a strong case in favour of Morton (as discoverer), but it is now acknowledged that the strongest claim to the title is that of Crawford Long."

Finally, to demonstrate further the opinion held around the world of Long and his work, this incident is related: Rev. Louie D. Newton, Atlanta Baptist minister, in 1946, was a member of a committee of seven invited to attend a meeting in Moscow, Russia. One of the members of this committee was a physician, and knowing Dr. Newton's interest in medical and surgical matters, invited him one morning to witness operations performed by the famed surgeon, Sergei

S. Yudin. After seeing two or three extensive chest operations, Dr. Newton met Dr. Yudin and found that he spoke perfect English. "Where are you from?" asked Yudin. "From Atlanta, Georgia," was the reply. "Ah," said the Russian, "Georgia, the home of the discoverer of anesthesia, Crawford Long."

The words of commendation and praise of Dr. Long, and the monuments erected to his memory are well deserved, but the discovery of anesthesia alone, as incomparable as it was, could not justify all the honors which have been heaped upon him. High character and ethical conduct played their part, without which the homage we pay him could not be so unalloyed. His modesty has annoyed us, and his reticence to act in his own behalf has disturbed our sleep, but to him is coming the glory which is his. When Long gains full possession of his rights, it may well be said, "Blessed are the meek."

Conclusion

The fact that Crawford Long administered the first surgical anesthetic, as described in the foregoing pages, is generally admitted. Few important scientific events are better attested by authentic documentary evidence. Most authors consider Long's accomplishment as the *discovery* of surgical anesthesia; others contend that the word "discovery" also must include the demonstration of something new to the world. While such an explanation is interesting, it is asking too much of one word. Henry Jacob Bigelow was one of Morton's staunchest advocates; and whoever first *suggested* anesthesia, Bigelow named Long as the *discoverer* when he declared, "He who verifies the suggestion is the true discoverer."[62]

Dr. Morton gave the first demonstration of surgical anesthesia before an audience destined to introduce it to the world; therefore, in order to show that Long's discovery was a vital factor in this momentous occasion, it is necessary to prove that Morton learned of successful ether anesthesia from Charles T. Jackson, and that Jackson learned of it from Long. The first fact seems to be granted, almost without a dissenting voice, while a large part of the chapter, "Ether Controversy Retold," is devoted in trying to prove the second fact. However much one may be convinced that Jackson's knowledge of the practical application of surgical anesthesia was obtained from Crawford Long, it is a difficult proposition to confirm after this lapse of years. Jackson's record for covetousness in matters of a similar nature furnishes reasonable ground for suspecting him of appropriating Long's discovery as his own, to accomplish which several easy and plausible opportunities have been described in detail.

The seven years Charles T. Jackson spent in the McLean Hospital as a mental case, from 1873 to 1880, are shrouded in secrecy. Efforts to ascertain whether he said, wrote, or did anything during that time which would shed further light upon the discovery of anesthesia have been unsuccessful. The authorities have refused to divulge anything. There may be nothing to tell, or there may be something of importance. Patients so unfortunately afflicted as Dr. Jackson may have lucid intervals when they can disclose facts upon which reliance may be placed. If anything worthwhile is revealed it is hoped that future writers may give it publication.

Many different and improved methods of anesthesia have been introduced since Long put James Venable asleep. Anesthesiology has become a well-established branch of medicine, and under the able leadership of those who are dedicating their careers to research in this field, still greater advances may be expected in the future. The simple way with sulphuric ether, however, continues to offer a satisfactory anesthetic, especially for children, and will not be entirely discarded. Many experienced anesthetists appear to bear a relieved look when they hear that ether anesthesia is requested for the patient. Certainly ether is the agent of choice for the occasional anesthetist, affording, as it does, unaided, not only safe relaxation and freedom from pain, but also what many patients ask for, loss of consciousness.

APPENDIX

first operation.

Atlanta DeKalb Co Ga.
   Winter 3rd 1853

C W Lingell D

It affords me pleasure to certify & I do hereby affirm that I saw & was present at an operation upon Mr James M Venable to wit the cutting out & removing of a Tumor from the neck of the said James M Venable.

The operation was performed when Mr Venable was under the *influence* of Sulphuric Ether, produced by inhaling the same. I was intimate with Mr Venable at the time of the operation; & afterwards frequently conversed with him upon the subject & he often told me that the operation produced no pain. The operation was performed in the Town of Jefferson Jackson County & State of Georgia in the year One Thousand Eight Hundred & Forty Two. Yours &c

Appendix

I Edmund S Rawls of the County of [Jones?] and state of Georgia, certify that during the year 1842 I resided at my father's in Jefferson Jackson County and that I was present and witnessed Dr. C. W. Long cut out one tumour from the back of Mr James Venable's neck and that he was under the influence of Sulphuric Ether when the operation was performed. Mr Venable did not show any sign of pain from the cutting and stated after the operation was over that he did not suffer the least degree of pain from the performance.

The wens were cut out at different times [during] the spring or summer of 1842. I [have] not [.....] [......] during both of the operations. I [frequently?] inhaled ether for its exhilerating effects and know that it was ether which was inhaled by Mr Venable when the operations were performed.

Sworn to and subscribed before me this fourth day of August 1853 —

F. A. Rawls [J.P.C.]

Edmund S. Rawls

Appendix

James Venable
                    To Dr. C. W. Long   Dr
1842.
January 28th Sulphuric Ether   25
March 30 Ether & Extracting Tumour 2.00
May 13 Sulphuric Ether   25
June 6 Extracting Tumour   2.00

Georgia
Jackson County   I P. F. Hinton
              Clerk of the
Superior Court of said County
do certify that the above account is a correct copy of an original
entry made in his Book for
Medical services for the year
1842.
    Given under my hand
& seal of office this 27th of March
1854.   P. F. Hinton, Clerk

Appendix

Appendix

I do certify that Dr Crawford W. Long of Jefferson, Jackson Co Ga advised my husband Dr Joseph B. Carlton, a resident of Athens, Ga to try sulphuric ether as an anesthetic in his practice.

In Nov or Dec 1844 in Jefferson Ga while on a visit to that place and in the office of Dr Long, my husband extracted a tooth from a boy who was under the influence by inhalation of sulphuric ether, without pain, the boy not knowing when it was done.

I further certify that the fact of Dr Long using sulphuric ether by inhalation to prevent pain was frequently spoken of in the county of Jackson at this time and was quite notorious.

      Mrs Emma B. Carlton

Sworn to and subscribed before me
June 29th 1907   Frank Betts
N. J. Allgood   N. P., Clarke County Ga.

REFERENCES

1. Emmet F. Horine, "Episodes in the History of Anesthesia," *Journal of the History of Medicine*, 1:4, October, 1946, p. 521.
2. John F. Fulton and Madeline E. Stanton, *The Centennial of Surgical Anesthesia, An Annotated Catalogue*. New York: Henry Schuman, 1946, p. 6.
3. H. J. Bigelow, *Congress Report, Ether Discovery*, 1852-1863.
4. Victor Robinson, *Victory Over Pain*. New York: Henry Schuman, 1946, pp. 28-30.
5. H. J. Bigelow, *loc. cit.*
6. *Ibid.*
7. Fulton and Stanton, *op. cit.*, p. 7.
8. Myra E. Babcock, "Brief Outline of History of Anesthesia," *Grace Hopkins Bulletin*, 10, April, p. 6-21.
9. Molly McQuaker, *Current Researches in Anesthesia and Analgesia*. VIII, 1. January-February, 1929, pp. 1-3.
10. Michael Faraday, "Effects of Inhaling the Vapors of Sulphuric Ether," *Quarterly Journal of Science and the Arts*, IV, 1818. pp. 158-159.
11. Jonathan Periera, *Elements of Materia Medica and Therapeutics*. Philadelphia: Lea & Blanchard, 1843.
12. H. B. Shafer, *American Medical Profession*, 1783-1850. New York: Columbia University Press, 1936, p. 140.
13. Logan Clendening, *Romance of Medicine*. Garden City, New York: Garden City Publishing Company, 1933, p. 308.
14. S. D. Gross, *Lives of Eminent American Physicians and Surgeons*. Philadelphia: Lindsey and Blakiston, 1861, p. 805.
15. J. C. Trent, "Surgical Anesthesia, 1846-1946," *Journal of the History of Medicine*, 1:4, October, 1946, pp. 505-514.
16. Valentine Mott, *Pain and Anesthesia*. Washington: McGill and Winterow, 1863.
17. Victor Robinson, *op. cit.*, p. 80.
18. Francis Long Taylor, *Crawford W. Long and the Discovery of Ether Anesthesia*. New York: Paul B. Hoeber, 1928.

I am indebted to Mrs. Taylor for most of the data concerning Dr. Long's early life and family.

19. Peter Robert, *The History of the Medical Department of Transylvania University*. Louisville: John P. Morton & Company, 1905. (Filson Club Publications No. 20.)
20. H. M. Lyman, *Artificial Anaesthesia and Anaesthetics*. New York: William Wood & Co., 1881, p. 6.
21. R. F. Stone, *Biography of Eminent American Physicians and Surgeons*. Indianapolis: Carlon & Hollenbeck, 1894, p. 89.
22. Robinson, *op. cit.*, p. 83.
23. August Schachner, *Ephraim McDowell*. Philadelphia: J. B. Lippincott Co., 1921, p. 62.
24. Joseph Krafka, Jr., "Long, Eve and Dugas: The Ether Controversy," *Journal of the Medical Association of Georgia*, xxxiii:11, Nov., 1944, pp. 330-334.

25. J. C. Warren, "Etherization, with Surgical Remarks," editorial in *Medical Record*, January 1947.
26. Seale Harris, *Banting's Miracle*. Philadelphia: J. B. Lippincott Co., 1946, p. 98.
27. J. Marion Sims, "Discovery of Anesthesia." *Virginia Medical Monthly*, IV:2, 1877, pp. 81-100.
28. Luther B. Grandy, "A Contribution to the History of the Discovery of Modern Surgical Anesthesia," *Virginia Medical Monthly*, XX:7, October 1893, pp. 577-588.
29. Hugh H. Young, "Long, the Discoverer of Anesthesia: A Presentation of the Original Documents," *Johns Hopkins Hospital Bulletin*, 1897, No. 8, pp. 174-184.
30. E. S. Ellis, *Ancient Anodynes*. London: Wm. Heinemann, 1946, p. 149.
31. Joseph Jacobs, *Dr. Crawford W. Long, the Distinguished Physician—Pharmacist*. Atlanta, 1919.
32. Hubert Royster, "Minor Surgery in Taboo," *Surgery*, August, 1939.
33. Evarts A. Graham, "Ether and Humbug," *Journal of the American Medical Association*, 133-2, Jan. 11, 1947, pp. 97-100.
34. Rudolph Matas, "Systemic or Cardiovascular Effects of Arteriovenous Fistulae," *Transactions of the Southern Surgical Association*, 1923, p. 663.
35. H. H. Branham, "Aneurysmal Varix of the Femoral Artery and Vein, etc.," *International Journal of Surgery*, New York, 1890, III, p. 250.
36. Curt Proskauer, "The Simultaneous Discovery of Rectal Anesthesia by Marc Dupuy and Nikolai Ivanovich Pirogoff," *Journal of the History of Medicine*, II:3, Summer 1947, pp. 379-384.
37. W. H. Welch, *Consideration of the Introduction of Surgical Anesthesia*. Boston: The Barta Press, 1908.
38. Harvey Cushing, *Life of William Osler*. Oxford: Clarendon Press, 1925, p. 604.
49. Atlanta *Constitution*, Jan. 17, 1921, p. 5.
40. George H. Bunch, "Doctor Charles Thomas Jackson," *Southern Medicine and Surgery*, 108-3, March 1946, pp. 63-68.
41. Victor Robinson, *Victory Over Pain*. New York: Henry Schuman, 1946, p. 135.
42. J. B. Woodworth, "Charles Thomas Jackson," *The American Geologist*, XX:2, August 1897, pp. 69-110.
43. Bunch, *loc. cit.*
44. S. I. Prime, *Life of Samuel F. B. Morse*, New York: Appleton & Co., 1875.
45. Carlton Mabee, *American Leonardo*. New York: Alfred A. Knopf, 1943.
46. Bunch, *loc. cit.*
47. Hugh H. Young, "Crawford W. Long, The Pioneer in Ether

References

Anesthesia," *Bulletin of the History of Medicine*, xii:2, July 1942, pp. 191-225.
48. Charles T. Jackson, *Manual of Etherization*. Boston: J. B. Mansfield, 1861.
49. Thomas E. Keys, *The History of Surgical Anesthesia*. New York: Henry Schuman, 1945, p. 23.
50. Woodworth, *op. cit.*, p. 95.
51. Howard Riley Raper, *Man Against Pain*. New York: Prentice-Hall, 1945, p. 113.
52. Robinson, *op. cit.*, p. 115.
53. Fulton and Stanton, *op. cit.*, p. 55.
54. Keys, *op. cit.*, p. 26.
55. Fielding H. Garrison, *History of Medicine*. Philadelphia: W. B. Saunders Co., 1921, p. 541.
56. Arturo Castiglioni, *History of Medicine*. New York: Alfred A. Knopf, 1941, p. 723.
57. Howard W. Haggard, *Doctor in History*. New Haven: Yale University Press, 1934, p. 348.
58. Samuel W. Lambert and George M. Goodwin, *Medical Leaders*. Indianapolis: The Bobbs-Merrill Co., 1929, p. 273.
59. John Homans, *Textbook of Surgery*, Sixth Edition. Springfield, Ill: Charles C. Thomas, 1945, p. 1128.
60. Chauncey D. Leake, "Historical Development of Surgical Anesthesia," *Scientific Monthly*, March 1925, pp. 304-328.
61. Douglas Guthrie, *History of Medicine*. Philadelphia: J. B. Lippincott Co., 1946, p. 304.
62. H. J. Bigelow, *Congress Reports*, p. 17.

BIBLIOGRAPHY

Abbott, J. H., "Discovery of Etherization," *Atlantic Monthly*, June 21, 1868, pp. 718-725.
Anesthesia Centennial Number, *Journal of the History of Medicine and Allied Sciences*, 1:4, Oct. 1946, St. Louis and New York: Henry Schuman.
Beaumont, *Life and Letters of William*. St. Louis and New York: C. V. Mosby Co., 1939.
Babcock, Myra E., "Brief Outline of the History of Anesthesia," *Grace Hopkins Bulletin*, April 1926.
Bigelow, H. J., "Insensibility During Surgical Operations Produced by Inhalation," *Boston Medical and Surgical Journal*, XXXV, Nov. 10, 1846, pp. 309-317.
Boland, F. K., "Crawford W. Long, the Discoverer of Anesthesia," *Southern Medical Journal*, XV:11, Nov. 1922, pp. 919-923.
———, "Centennial of Crawford Long's First Use of Ether in Surgery," *Surgery*, XIII:2, Feb. 1943, pp. 270-281.
Bunch, G. H., "Doctor Charles Thomas Jackson," *Southern Medicine and Surgery*, 198, March 1946, pp. 63-65.
Buxton, D. W., "Crawford Williamson Long (1815-1878), the Pioneer of Anesthesia and the First to Suggest and Employ Ether Inhalation During Surgical Operations," *Proceedings of the Royal Society of Medicine*, Section 5, 1912, pp. 19-45.
Castiglioni, A.A., *History of Medicine*. New York: Alfred A. Knopf. 1941.
———, "Centenary of Sulphurous Ether as an Inhaled Anesthetic," *Medical Record*. 160, Jan. 1947, pp. 39-40.
———, "Century of Ether Anesthesia." Editorial, *Review of Gastroenterology*, 13:5, Sept.-Oct. 1946, pp. 384-385.
Chiles, Rosa P., "Dr. Crawford W. Long, Discoverer of Anesthesia," *Munsey's Magazine*, 45, 1911, pp. 623-630.
Clendening, Logan, *Romance of Medicine: Behind The Doctor*. Garden City, New York: Garden City Publishing Co., 1933.
———, "One Hundred Years of Anesthesia," *Hygeia, A.M.A.*,

XX-4, April 1942, p. 274, *et seq*.
———, "Literature and Material on Anesthesia in the Library of Medical History of the University of Kansas School of Medicine, *Kansas Bulletin of the Medical Library*, 33, Jan. 1945, pp. 123-138.
Crenshaw, Hansell, "Conquest of Pain, *"Uncle Remus's The Home Magazine*, XXV, May 1909, pp. 7-9, 17.
Cutler, Max, "Contributions of Crawford Long and His Contemporaries to American Medicine," *Journal of the Medical Association of Georgia*, XXV:3, March 1936, pp. 75-81.
DaCosta, J. C., *Papers and Speeches*. Philadelphia: W. B. Saunders Co., 1931.
Dana, R. H., Jr. "History of the Ether Discovery: Report of the Trustees of the Massachusetts General Hospital, *Littell's Living Age*, 16, March 18, 1848, pp. 529-571.
Davy, Humphry, *Researches, Chemical and Philosophical, Chiefly Concerning Nitrous Oxide, or Dephlogisticated Nitrous Air and Its Respiration*. London: J. Johnson, 1800.
Duncum, Barbara M., *Development of Inhalation Anesthesia*. Oxford: Oxford University Press, 1947.
Ellis, E. S., *Ancient Anodynes*. London: William Heinemann, 1946.
Emerson, E. W., "History of the Gift of Painless Surgery," *Atlantic Monthly*, 78, Nov. 1946, pp. 679-686.
Faraday, Michael, "Effects of Inhaling the Vapors of Sulphuric Ether, *"Quarterly Journal of Science and the Arts*, 4, 1818, pp. 158-159.
Fitz, Reginald, "Value of Imponderables," *New England Journal of Medicine*. 236: 16, April 17, 1947, pp. 555-562.
Flagg, P. J., *Art of Anesthesia*, Philadelphia: J. B. Lippincott Co., 1939.
Flexner, J. T., *Doctors on Horseback*. New York: Viking Press, 1937.
Fulop-Miller, Rene: *Triumph Over Pain*. New York: Literary Guild of America, 1938.

Fulton, J. F., "Crawford W. Long," *Dictionary of American Biography*. New York: Charles Scribner's Sons, 1933, XI, pp. 623-630.

Fulton, J. F. and Stanton, Madeline, *Centennial of Surgical Anesthesia, An Annotated Catalogue*, New York: Henry Schuman, 1946.

Garrison, F. H., *Introduction to the History of Medicine*. Philadelphia: W. B. Saunders Co., 1929.

Gay, Martin, *Statement of the Claims of Charles T. Jackson, M.D., to the Discovery of the Applicability of Sulphuric Ether to the Prevention of Pain in Surgical Operations*. Boston: David Clapp, 1847.

Goss, I. H., "Long and His Discovery," *Atlanta Journal-Record of Medicine*, X, Nov. 1908, pp. 401-409.

Grandy, L. B., "Contribution to the History of the Discovery of Modern Surgical Anesthesia," *Virginia Medical Monthly*, XX:7, Oct., 1893, pp. 577-588.

———, "Discovery of Anesthesia, and the Alleged Relations between Dr. C. W. Long and Dr. P. A. Wilhite," *New York Medical Journal*, July 20, 1895, pp. 79-81.

Gross, S. D., *Lives of Eminent American Physicians and Surgeons*. Philadelphia: Lindsey & Blakiston, 1861.

Guthrie, Douglas, *History of Medicine*. Philadelphia: J. B. Lippincott Co., 1946, p. 304.

Gwathmey, J. T., *Anesthesia*. New York: D. Appleton Co., 1914.

Haggard, H. W., *Doctor in History*. New Haven: Yale University Press, 1934, pp. 344-354.

Hickman, H. H., *Letter on Suspended Animation Containing Experiments Showing That It May Be Safely Employed On Animals with the View of Ascertaining Its Probable Utility in Surgical Operations on the Human Subject*. Ironbridge: W. Smith, 1824.

Jackson, C. T., *Manual of Etherization*, Boston: J. B. Mansfield, 1861.

Jacobs, Joseph, *Dr. Crawford W. Long, the Distinguished Physician-Pharmacist. Some Personal Recollections and Private Correspondence of Dr. Crawford Williamson Long, Discoverer of Anesthesia with Sulphuric Ether, Together with Documentary Proofs of His Priority in This Wonderful Discovery*. Atlanta, 1919.

Jirka, F. J., *American Doctors of Destiny*. Chicago: Black Cat Press, 1940.

Johnson, C. B., "Lest We Forget, or Dr. Crawford W. Long, the First Anesthetist," *Illinois Medical Journal*, 32, Aug. 1917, pp. 122-129.

Jones, L. H., "Crawford W. Long and His Discovery," *Transactions of the Medical Association of Georgia*, 50 1899, pp. 375-388.

Keys, T. E., *History of Surgical Anesthesia*. New York: Henry Schuman, 1945.

Krafka, Joseph, Jr., "Long, Eve and Dugas," *Journal of the Medical Association of Georgia*, XXXIII:11, Nov. 1944, pp. 330-334.

Lambert, S. W. and Goodwin, G. W., *Medical Leaders*. Indianapolis: Bobbs-Merrill Co., 1927.

Leake, C. D., "Historical Development of Surgical Anesthesia," *Scientific Monthly*, 20, March 1925, pp. 304-328.

Long, C. W., "Account of the First Use of Sulphuric Ether by Inhalation as an Anesthetic in Surgical Operations," *Southern Medical and Surgical Journal*, 5, Dec. 1849, pp. 705-713.

Long, J. W., "Crawford W. Long, the Discoverer of Ether Anesthesia, *Transactions of the Southern Surgical Association, XXXVII*, 1924, pp. 312-324.

Lord, J. L. & H. C., "Defense of Charles T. Jackson's Claim to the Discovery of Etherization," *Littell's Living Age*, Boston, 1848.

Lundy, J. S., "Crawford W. Long Day Address, University of Georgia, March 30, 1943," *Journal of the Medical Association of Georgia*, 32, May, 1943, pp. 167-172.

Lyman, H. M., *Artificial Anesthesia and Anesthetics*. New York: William Wood & Co., 1881.

Magruder, E. M., "Discovery of Surgical Anesthesia," *Virginia Medical Semi-Monthly*, 1915, 41, 554-559, 577-582, 608-614; 42, 12-16.

McGill, R. C., "Progress in Anesthesia, Reply to L. A. Wassersug," *American Mercuy*, 60, March, 1945, p. 376.

Merrill, G. P. and Fulton, J. F., "Charles T. Jackson," *Dictionary of American Biography*. New York: Charles Scribner's Sons, 1932, IX pp. 536-538.

Mettler, C. C., *History of Medicine*, Philadelphia: Blakiston Company, 1947.

Meyer, Jesse Shipe, *Life and Letters of Dr. William Beaumont*. St. Louis: C. V. Mosby Company, 1912.

Minder, W. G., *Dr. Crawford W. Long, the Discoverer of Ether as an Anesthetic*. Atlanta, 1940.

Moore, James, *Method of Preventing or Diminishing Pain in Several Operations in Surgery*. London: T. Cadill, 1784.

Morton, W. G.,* "Invention of Anesthetic Inhalation, or Discovery of Anesthesia." *Virginia Medical Monthly*, VI:12, March 1880, pp. 949-985.

Morton, W. T. G., *Memoir to the Academy of Science at Paris on a New Use of Sulphuric Ether*. Presented in 1847. New York: Henry Schuman, 1946.

Morton, W. T. G., *Statements, Supported by Evidence, of W. T. G. Morton, M.D., on His Claim to the Discovery of the Anesthetic Properties of Ether*. Washington, 1853.

Mott, Valentine, *Pain and Anesthesia*, Washington: McGill and Winterow, 1863.

Packard, F. R., *History of Medicine in the United States*. New York, 1931.

Paget, Sir James, "Escape From Pain: History of a Discovery," *Eclectic Magazine*, 94, February 1880, pp. 219-228.

* Son of W. T. G. Morton.

———, "Painless Operations in Surgery by the Use of Etherization." (Reprinted from North British Review) *Littell's Living Age.* 13, June 12, 1847, pp. 481-496.

Pennsylvania, University of, "Account of the Ceremonies of the Unveiling of a Bronze Medallion in the Medical Building, March 30, 1912, to the Memory of Crawford W. Long, of the Class of 1839," Bulletin of the University, 1912.

Quillian, G. W., "Crawford W. Long," *Journal of the Medical Association of Georgia*, 10, July, 1921, p. 543.

Raper, H. R., *Man Against Pain.* New York: Prentice-Hall, 1945.

Rice, N. P., *Trials of a Public Benefactor*, New York: Pudney and Russell, 1858.

Robinson, J. Ben, "William T. G. Morton and Ether," *Journal of the American Dental Association*, 33:23, December 1, 1946, pp. 1572-1576.

Robinson, Victor, *Victory Over Pain.* New York: Henry Schuman, 1946.

Shafer, H. B., *American Medical Profession, 1783-1850.* New York: Columbia University Press, 1936.

Sims, J. M., "Discovery of Anesthesia," *Virginia Medical Monthly*, IV:2, May 1877, pp. 81-100.

Smith, A. J., "Documentary Evidence Bearing Upon Crawford W. Long's Discovery of Ether Anesthesia, with Seventeen Photostatic Reproductions of the Most Important Documents," "*Old Penn.*" Weekly Review of the University of Pennsylvania, XIV:1, Oct. 2, 1915, pp. 27-44.

Smith, Truman, *Inquiry Into The Origin of Modern Anesthesia.* Hartford: Brown and Gross, 1867.

Snyder, Mrs. E. E., *Biology In The Making.* New York: McGraw-Hill Book Company, 1940.

Stone, R. F., *Biography of Eminent Physicians and Surgeons.* Indianapolis: Carlon and Hollenbeck, 1914.

Bibliography 159

Stuart, H. L., *Crawford W. Long, a Biographical Sketch of the World's Greatest Benefactor.* New York, 1879.

Taylor, Mrs. F. L. "Crawford Williamson Long," *Annals of Medical History*, VII, 1925, pp. 267-296 and pp. 394-424.

———, *Crawford W. Long and the Discovery of Ether Anesthesia.* New York: Paul B. Hoeber, 1928.

Underwood, E. A., "Before and After Morton," *British Medical Journal*, Oct. 12, 1926, pp. 525-531.

U. S. Congress Reports, "Ether Discovery, 1852-1863." From the Library of John Farquhar Fulton.

U. S. Congress, First Session, 1925-1926. "Proceedings in Statuary Hall of the United States Capitol upon Unveiling and Presentation of the Statue of Crawford W. Long, by the State of Georgia, March 30, 1926." Washington: Government Printing Office, 1926.

Warren, J. C., *Etherization with Surgical Remarks.* Boston: W. D. Ticknor and Co., 1848.

Wassersug, L. A., "One Hundred Years of Anesthesia," *American Mercury*, 60, Jan. 1945, pp. 114-119.

Welch, W. H., *Consideration of the Introduction of Surgical Anesthesia.* Boston: Barta Press, 1908.

Wellcome Historical Medical Museum, London, "Souvenir, Henry Hill Hickman," *Centenary Exhibition, 1830-1930.* London: Wellcome Foundation, 1930.

Wells, Horace, *History of the Discovery of the Application of Nitrous Oxide Gas, Ether and Other Vapors, to Surgical Operations.* Hartford: J. Gaylord Wells, 1847.

Williams, H. S., "Semicentennial of the Discovery of Anesthesia," *Harper's Weekly*, 40, Oct. 17, 1896, pp. 1031-1033.

———, "Century's Progress in Scientific Medicine," *Harper's New Monthly Magazine*, 99, June 1899, pp. 38-52.

Woodworth, J. B., "Charles Thomas Jackson," *American Geologist*, XX:2, Aug. 1897, pp. 66-110.

Young, H. H., "Long, the Discoverer of Anesthesia: Presentation of His Original Documents," *Johns Hopkins Hospital Bulletin*, 8, 1897, pp. 174-184.

——, "Crawford W. Long, the Pioneer in Ether Anesthesia," *Bulletin of the History of Medicine*, XII:2, July 1942, pp. 191-225.

www.ingramcontent.com/pod-product-compliance
Lightning Source LLC
Chambersburg PA
CBHW032025230426
43671CB00005B/208